T0285046

THE BLACK WIDOW

THE BLACK WIDOW

A Memoir

JEANETTE LEE
WITH DANA BENBOW

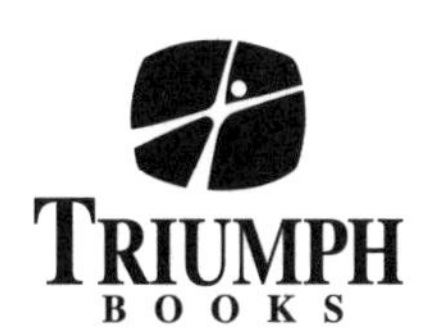

Library of Congress Cataloging-in-Publication Data

Names: Lee, Jeanette, author. | Benbow, Dana, author.
Title: The Black Widow : a memoir / Jeanette Lee with Dana Benbow.
Description: Chicago, Illinois : Triumph Books, 2024.
Identifiers: LCCN 2024002424 (print) | LCCN 2024002425 (ebook) | ISBN 9781637273999 (cloth) | ISBN 9781637275603 (pdf) | ISBN 9781637275610 (epub)
Subjects: LCSH: Lee, Jeanette. | Women pool players—United States—Biography. | Korean American women—Biography. | Scoliosis—Patients—United States—Biography. | Cancer—Patients—United States—Biography
Classification: LCC GV892.2.L44 A3 2024 (print) | LCC GV892.2.L44 (ebook) | DDC 794.73/3092 [B]—dc23/eng/20240229
LC record available at https://lccn.loc.gov/2024002424
LC ebook record available at https://lccn.loc.gov/2024002425

This book is available in quantity at special discounts for your group or organization. For further information, contact:

Triumph Books LLC
814 North Franklin Street
Chicago, Illinois 60610
(312) 337-0747
www.triumphbooks.com

Printed in U.S.A.

ISBN: 978-1-63727-399-9
Design by Nord Compo

All photos courtesy of the author unless otherwise indicated.

DEDICATION

MOM, I DEDICATE MY MEMOIR TO YOU. I could not have overcome what I have, let alone shared my story, if it were not for your unconditional love, your strength, your courage, your generosity to others, your hard work ethic, your grace, your strong will, your dedication and commitment to us, your girls, and to our entire family.

I watched you work so hard for everything you have, truly for our sake, Doris and mine, yet you were always ready to help anyone else, not for credit, but to acknowledge that God is good.

You always found a way to make time to help others, but who was there for you? Nobody. Your parents died while we were still young. The more I get to know you, the more I marvel at your courage, your strength, and your goodness.

I still marvel at the fact that you survived raising me. Whenever anyone gives me credit for working hard or being good to others, I give all the credit to you. I know that the best things about me are the things I've learned from you.

I got to watch you firsthand, and it kills me that I took it so for granted. I'm so blessed because of you. Your faith in God and your courage to keep going, no matter how tough things got, inspired me to work hard for what I wanted, and to never give up.

You made yourself a servant of God, and you never complained. I remember all the times you asked, "Jeanette, who is your neighbor? Love your neighbor as yourself." Every time I was proud of this or that accomplishment, you would say, "Remember, be humble and kind." All of that, all of you, had its impact on me, and I'm so proud to say I learned it from you.

You managed to stay humble, in spite of all you've accomplished, and still today, you continue to try to improve yourself for the benefit of others. What a role model you have been to me and anyone whose life you have touched.

You have been everything to me, even when you were not there, you actually were there. In my heart and being. It's just taken me a long time to recognize that.

It was the foundation that you built that gave me the wings to fly, the courage to endure, and the strength to never give up.

As with all my children and grandchildren, Mom, I love you to the moon and back, to infinity and beyond, forever and ever, no matter what. Without you, this book would not have been possible.

—Jeanette Lee

CONTENTS

FOREWORD

THE FIRST TIME I MET JEANETTE LEE, I saw what everybody else in the world saw—except for Jeanette Lee. I saw this wicked, badass, athletic woman at the pool table, who clearly didn't think she was any of those things.

Jeanette is, and always has been, a humble woman. She is also a woman who, through the unimaginable pain of scoliosis, countless emotional and physical obstacles, and relentless, persistent hard work, became a billiards superstar.

But she is a woman who never thought of herself as a superstar. What Jeanette didn't know, and everybody else in the world knew, was that she was remarkable, too. And she absolutely deserved to be talked about in the same conversations as other great athletes.

As she took to the green felt tables in tournaments, exuding The Black Widow persona, she trounced her opponents. She rose to become the No. 1 women's pool player in the world just five years after she walked into a billiards hall as a skinny, lost, 18-year-old rebel searching for a purpose in life.

Jeanette scratched and clawed her way to a meteoric rise, to pool stardom, and she did it wearing all-black, edgy outfits, with a swagger that made everyone think she must be the most confident woman in the world.

She was confident when she was playing pool, but Jeanette wasn't confident off the table. Jeanette was, and is, an inspiration to so many people, including me.

The reality is that other superstar athletes were incredibly impressed with what Jeanette was doing. She wasn't just succeeding in a woman's sport. She was making waves in an individual sport that was dominated by men. And she was winning.

Jeanette was exactly the type of female athlete I had in mind when I founded the Women's Sports Foundation in 1974. And 20 years later, when I met Jeanette, I knew she would be a perfect ambassador for our cause.

In 1994, Jeanette received a call from the late Yolanda Jackson, who was head of athlete engagement at our foundation, and she was invited to attend our Annual Salute Dinner in New York City. That was the beginning of her long-lasting involvement and love for the foundation.

"They showed genuine concern for my future, and I felt I had an instant family of the most positive people I had ever met," Jeanette said in 1994. "Since then, I have dedicated myself to being the best person, sportswoman, leader, and role model that I can be. None of us ever succeeds totally in achieving these goals, but the continuing influence of the Women's Sports Foundation is invaluable to all of us in our journey toward them."

Jeanette went on to serve on our board from 2001 to 2006, serving two back-to-back three-year terms as the trustee of the foundation.

Jeanette was always a fierce advocate for women, not just in sports, but in life. She has always been very concerned, and always willing to help in any way she could to forward the cause of women in sports. She cares deeply about equal pay, equal access, and working toward giving women the honor and recognition they deserve.

Among the advocates for women's equality in sports, Jeanette is a leader.

At the height of her career in the late 1990s and 2000s, *Sports Illustrated* went to major cities in America and polled the public, trying to gauge name recognition among the athletes of the day. More than 60 percent of the people polled knew the name Jeanette Lee, or The Black Widow, and associated it with the sport of pool. Not only did she beat the greatest male pool player in the world, Efren Reyes, who registered less than 1 percent name recognition, she took the sport to new heights.

Jeanette is an incredible outlier, a woman who gained stature in a niche sport, and as she rose to fame at the pool table, she transcended her sport to become an American icon. She is the only woman billiards player in America to land a major deal outside of the sport. And she landed some major deals, including well-known companies like ESPN, Ford, Canadian Club, Frontgate, Reebok, and Bass Pro Shops.

Just stop for a moment and think about everything Jeanette Lee has accomplished in her sport. She has won every major title in billiards, more than 30 national and international titles, including the WPBA Nationals, the U.S. Open, the 1999 Bar Table World Championship, and a gold medal at the 2001 World Games in Akita, Japan. She was the WPBA Sportsperson of the Year, earned Player of the Year honors from both *Billiards Digest* and *Pool & Billiard* magazine, was the 2004 International Trick Shot champion, and took home back-to-back Empress Cup titles in 2008 and 2009.

She has been inducted into three different halls of fame, the Billiard Congress of America and WPBA Hall of Fame in 2013, and the Asian Hall of Fame in 2015, which wasn't just about sports. It was about stardom. She is in the Asian Hall of Fame alongside people like Bruce Lee, I.M. Pei, Connie Chung, Daniel Dae Kim, Carrie Ann Inaba, and Kristi Yamaguchi.

Just think about what Jeanette meant to not only the sport of billiards but to all athletes. Just think about her fight and her perseverance.

There are, after all, so many young Jeanette Lees out there in this world, just waiting for their turn, fighting for their chance to become star athletes. And some day, they will have their own story to tell.

Jeanette Lee has one of the most inspiring life stories you will ever read.

—Billie Jean King
International Tennis Hall of Famer,
winner of 39 Grand Slam titles,
and recipient of the Presidential Medal of Freedom

CHAPTER 1

PLUNGING OFF A CLIFF STRAIGHT INTO THE ARMS OF POOL

I WAS A SKINNY, ashamed, insecure, 18-year-old girl when I walked into Chelsea Billiards, a mystical club in New York City full of pompous businessmen, raucous hustlers, arrogant yuppies, and far more glamour than I ever dreamed a pool hall could have.

I was nothing more than a rebellious teenager searching for a purpose in life when I fell in love with green felt tables, colorful pool balls, and the intense aura of edgy competition mixed with pure class.

Chelsea Billiards served cappuccinos at the front desk. There were workers wearing crisp, collared shirts and sharply pleated pants, bustling around, emptying out beautifully engraved, charcoal ashtrays.

Chelsea was a 15,000-square-foot, enchanting pool mecca in Lower Manhattan, open 24 hours a day. It was massive, taking up two floors and boasting more than 55 tables. Around those tables were shady hustlers, aggressive gamblers, terrible players, and absolutely incredible players.

The pool halls I had been to before with my high school boyfriend as a runaway teen were dark, seedy, musty places that served hot dogs, chips, and cheap coffee. The atmosphere was gritty, and the jukebox blared heavy metal.

As the men played inside those dank halls, they would stare lewdly at my teenage body, mumbling inappropriate comments as they smirked, giving each other knowing looks.

Those men were clumsy with their cue sticks, their shots weren't clean, and it seemed as if they were just banging the balls as hard as they could so they could grunt in victory. The whole place reeked of overpowering masculinity.

When I walked into Chelsea Billiards at 18 years old in 1989, after working my shift at a Korean computer company five blocks away, I was blown away. I fell in love with pool, and I fell hard.

Chelsea Billiards had just opened with a ritzy, grand celebration and my friend was talking about this amazing wonderland filled with green felt tables that seemed to go on forever.

They talked about the incredible skill of the players, and the hustlers who downplayed their talents to the newcomers they called "fish." The hustlers would bait those fish and walk away each night with wads of cash stuffed into their front pockets.

Maybe pool didn't have to be a cheap dive full of unsavory characters. Maybe it didn't have to be a dark and seedy sport. Maybe pool could be captivating, edgy, and beautiful.

After hearing my friend talk about this billiards haven, I couldn't finish my shift fast enough. When the clock struck 5:00 PM, I bolted out and headed to 54 W. 21st Street in New York City to check this place out.

I had no idea, really, what I was doing there. But I look back now, and I know I was searching for something that made sense in my life. Something that made me feel like I belonged. Something that gave me purpose.

In 1989, I was a lost, floundering soul. I was an 18-year-old wannabe rebel, desperately grasping for something that made me feel worthy.

I had never really fit in. I had always been the outcast, no matter where I was, no matter what I was doing, and no matter who I was with. That is a lonely, gut-wrenching, and isolating feeling.

Growing up, I was the youngest of two daughters, with an overachieving sister who I never felt I quite measured up to. Doris was two years older than me, and she was so sensible, so pretty, so smart, and she had this shiny, long hair that she always parted to one side.

Her body was thin and flat-chested like mine but she looked great in jeans and she seemed totally comfortable in her own body. She had no problem wearing fitted shirts, whereas I would wear loose shirts and stuff my bra, hoping I looked like I had breasts, but at the same time, I was hoping no one would notice my chest. I loved the clothes she wore and the music she listened to.

I was a 13-year-old girl on the brink of puberty who was diagnosed with severe scoliosis, who was forced to wear a clunky, full-body, plastic brace that made me feel like Frankenstein. It was itchy and uncomfortable and it would chafe my skin until I was raw with blisters.

I had to walk into school wearing a pair of men's size 3X jogging pants, big enough to cover the brace. And I had to wear a shirt that would reach high enough on my neck to hide the color of the brace, which was supposed to match my skin but didn't at all. I heard the bullies' taunts and the muffled laughter as I lumbered down the school halls. I saw the look of pity on the faces of nicer classmates as I walked to my desk.

The brace wasn't the only thing I was teased about. I was Korean American. I was repeatedly asked, not so nicely, if I was Bruce Lee's daughter or if I knew kung fu. The kids at school would chant, "ching chong chally wong" as I walked by, along with other ethnic slurs used to mock people of Asian descent. They used them to mock me, and it pissed me off. I also got bullied about my thick glasses, with kids knocking them off my face and calling me "Four Eyes" or "Bug Eyes." I couldn't help but get into fights sometimes, which I always lost because I was so puny.

I would go home after school to a towering co-op apartment building in the Crown Heights neighborhood of Brooklyn where I grew up, where almost all the families were Black. I was so jealous of those girls with their bodies that curved. I would sometimes wear two or three leggings under my jeans to make my thighs look thicker, and put socks in my bra to look bustier.

I was so skinny, so concave. When I put my feet together, you could see a gap between my thighs. I would walk into my homeroom in seventh grade and hear the chants, "Fall into the Gap," like the Gap commercial jingle at the time. There were rumors that I was a slut, and that I had the gap between my thighs because I was having sex with all the boys.

At home, I hated my parents' rules and the strict regimen. After I took a bath or shower, I was required to get down on my knees and scrub the tub. There was a time set to get homework done, brush my teeth, and go to bed.

Sleeping in wasn't allowed, even on Saturdays when there was no school, and I loved sleeping in. I remember as a teenager being so angry and frustrated, and screaming, "Mom, why won't you just leave me alone?" She told me I was wasting my life away in my bed, that I needed to be awake when the world was awake.

I ran away too many times to count, crashing on couches of whatever friend or teacher would take me in. I smoked cigarettes and marijuana, and I tried cocaine and acid. I took needles and jabbed them into my lobes making homemade pierced ears. I took a razor blade once and cut my forearm repeatedly so that a friend and I could be blood sisters. It took 28 slashes before my forearm started bleeding. I thought maybe my close friendship with her would make life better.

But nothing made life better. Nothing, it seemed, would ever take away the loneliness of feeling like an outcast.

> "Jeanette always wondered why she couldn't be understood. And she always searched for ways to make sense of that."
> —Doris Lee, Jeanette's sister

As I stood outside Chelsea Billiards in 1989, I still don't know what gave 18-year-old Jeanette Lee the courage to walk in. It was an intimidating place and, as I walked through that pool hall, I saw the men glancing my way.

But this time, they weren't staring at me lewdly. They were eying me with looks on their faces that seemed to say, "What is this skinny Asian girl doing here?"

I kind of wondered about that myself. I knew, deep down, my mom would hate what I was doing, her youngest daughter walking into a pool hall alone. I heard her voice echoing in my head: "This is not ladylike, Jeanette. This is not what I worked so hard for you to become."

I didn't care. I didn't want a life of mundane, everyday routine. That wasn't what raged in my soul.

I have never once been sorry I walked into that Lower Manhattan pool hall, nervous and out of my element. I never regretted making my way to the far back corner of the room where I saw a man named George Mikula practicing alone. He was the most graceful person I had ever seen. As he moved toward his next shot, it seemed as if his body was floating above the ground.

The club was loud and crowded but, as Mikula played, all the noise and people disappeared. It was like he and I were inside that pool hall alone, and our hearts were beating as one. I was so in tune with what he was doing, it felt almost dreamlike.

He would lean over and shoot, and he would make the cue ball dance. He had speed control, and he could make the cue ball go exactly where he wanted it to. He made pool look so unbelievably easy. His cue seemed like it was an extension of his arm. I was mesmerized.

As I watched Mikula create geometric magic on the table that night, something inside of me lit up, something I had never felt before. It was like being jolted awake from a very deep sleep. I later found out that he was one of the best straight pool players in the country.

I stayed that night for hours watching the men play, most who were old enough to be my father, and many who were old enough to be my grandfather. I loved the way they shattered the rack of balls, the way they lined up their next shot, and the creativity they showed playing patterns in their own personal style. I soaked it all in, and I couldn't get enough.

> "Jeanette told me she was drawn to pool that very first night at Chelsea Billiards, and it pulled her in like some magnetic force. It was like the world around her stopped, and there was nothing else but pool."
>
> —Tom George, Lee's longtime manager

I left Chelsea Billiards late that night and walked home alone with one thought invading my entire being: I had to learn to play pool like those guys played pool.

Then I started going to Chelsea Billiards every night.

I would bolt out of the office at 5:00 PM and practically run down the sidewalks, darting between the mob of New York City office workers leaving for the day. I would forget to eat as I practiced, sometimes repeating the same shot hundreds of times in a row until I got it just right. I didn't mind the hunger pangs, but I knew I had to eat.

There was a deli just around the corner from Chelsea that served custom-made sandwiches. I never wanted to waste minutes waiting in line to have a sandwich made, so I went to the crocks of soup. I would dip a cup of chicken noodle or vegetable beef, I would grab a baguette, and I would race back to the pool hall as quickly as I could.

I remember how annoyed I would get that I had to stop for food. I hated taking breaks, even going to the bathroom. All of it was a waste of precious time that I could be hitting balls.

On the weekends, I would wake up early in the morning inside my apartment at 23rd Street and Lexington Avenue in a panic, after a late night at Chelsea Billiards. I couldn't get back to the tables soon enough.

Many mornings, I would hop in a cab, even though the pool hall was only a few blocks away, about a 15–20-minute walk. I was sure going by taxi would get me there faster than walking. Even if it only saved me one or two minutes, that was one or two more minutes playing pool.

And I had to get back to the tables. I had to play as much as I could.

The men at Chelsea Billiards never acted like I was a nuisance or a bother. They were nice to me, some even practiced with me, but I learned that if I wanted any of them to play pool with me, I'd have to gamble with them. At the very least, they'd insist we play for table-time bill. As much pool as I was playing, at $15 per hour for two players, the table-time bill could be close to $100!

That's when I learned the art of negotiation. I didn't have much money at that age, so it was important that I win whenever I played. People have asked me for years if I ever hustled any guys playing pool and I'd say, "I didn't have to. Being a woman *was* the hustle." It was so easy for me to negotiate winning matches because I could assess someone's skill against mine as it really was. For most men, they just saw a woman. They just couldn't imagine that a woman could beat them playing pool. They recognized how hard I was working and how fast I was improving. I wasn't just some silly girl hanging around trying to get attention. I was serious.

Of course, I was still a girl, so there were plenty of guys trying to show me how to hold the cue. And every time I missed a shot, they were eager to teach me what to do next.

I finally felt what I had craved for so long. I started to fit in. I wasn't an outsider.

I had their respect. I had a purpose.

For the next three years, I scratched and clawed my way to become an elite athlete, climbing to the top of the sport of pocket billiards, despite the barriers and the naysayers around every corner.

I became the woman who devoured almost every opponent that came my way, eating them up and spitting them out like a black widow spider. I became known as "The Black Widow" of billiards.

My mother hated that nickname. She started flying to some of my pro events. She'd sit in the stands, watching my match, and then gently lean over to sweetly tell fans, opponents, managers—anyone who would listen—that my "Black Widow" nickname had been changed, and they should now call her daughter "The Lily of the Valley." Can you believe that didn't stick?

> "I did not like it. My sweet, beautiful daughter is not The Black Widow. Jeanette is like a lily to me. Jeanette didn't like it either, because of the negative image. But at some point, she had no choice but to accept it."
>
> —Sonja Lee, Jeanette's mother

I did hate the nickname "The Black Widow" at first. But to be honest, I ended up loving that moniker. I was, after all, the woman who wore black, shaking up the billiards fashion scene, which at that point was comprised of conservative silk blouses and pleated slacks. They all looked like they were going to work in an office.

I fought the icy glares from female opponents who couldn't understand why I had to look sexy as I played their sport. I was told more than once that I was not liked by the women, that they were incredibly jealous of me. It made me so sad because since I was a little girl, all I've ever wanted was to be liked, to have friends. I was never disrespectful. I had the reputation of being too cocky but how would they know? They didn't even give me a chance. They hated the attention I was getting. Yes, I was determined to be the best—I was confident—but that didn't mean I didn't respect them. Quite the opposite. I wasn't confident that I was better than them. I was confident that I would become the top-ranked woman in the world because I planned to work harder and smarter than anyone I'd ever seen and I had the rest of my life to prove it. But I was always respectful. I admired the top women pros and they treated me like dirt. They could've chosen to mentor me, teach me, guide me. I tried so hard to fit in.

When I made money, I tried buying slacks and blouses similar to theirs. That only lasted one match. I felt like I had a straitjacket on. I was so uncomfortable. "Here I go again," I told myself, "being a wannabe, not fitting in, misunderstood, and hated."

After playing awful and losing my first match, I decided I had to be me. No matter what, I had to stay true to who I was. I can't be my best self if I'm not being myself. I was from New York, where wearing black is very common, and I had style. I didn't know that, but I found out by all the attention I was getting. Back then, there was a strict dress code and I had terrible back pain all the time so it's not like I was wearing high heels or anything low cut. The women thought I was just getting attention because I was pretty. The truth of the matter is, if you can't win a match, nobody cares how pretty you are.

My longtime manager, Tom George, always told people the women didn't hate me. They hated the *idea* of me. I wasn't just walking into tournaments wearing fitted shirts, I was destroying the competition.

I had long black hair, long nails, and I wore red lipstick. I was sexy, even if I wasn't trying to be sexy, and the women players thought I was bad for the sport.

But I wasn't bad for the sport. I was good for the sport.

I turned the world of pocket billiards upside down, rising to the No. 1 pool player in the world by the time I was 23. I always thought I would be a much better player by the time I became No. 1 in the world. I still had so much to improve. That's when I realized, I needed to become the greatest I could be, not set my standards against others.

> "I was always impressed at how confident Jeanette was, on and off the table. You could tell right away she was in her element whenever she walked through the door. To see a beautiful Asian woman like her was very strange for most people so they didn't know how to react or feel about it. She brought an element that had never been seen before. She was beautiful, sexy, super confident, and super talented on the table. That intimidated a lot of people."
> —Tony Robles, one of the world's elite billiard champions

When I was at my peak, dominating the women's pool circuit, it felt like the media was in love with me. I couldn't understand that. I couldn't comprehend why I was so popular.

Tantalizing headlines flashed. Broadcasts blared: "A pool shark who wears an icy glare and distinctive black clothing while devouring her opponents. She is Jeanette Lee, The Black Widow of billiards."

I was on the covers of *Billiards Digest* and *Asian Week*, written about in *Sports Illustrated* articles, including one titled "Kiss of the Spider Woman," and featured in *USA Today*, *Forbes*, *People*, *Esquire*, *ESPN the Magazine*, *Shape*, *Maxim*, *Cigar Aficionado*, and *The New York Times*, all while I was a star on ESPN.

One reporter from *Muscle and Fitness* magazine, noting my menacing look at the table, asked what was I thinking when I'm down shooting. I went on and on about how much I loved being there, getting to play all these women whose billiard matches I had saved up and bought Accu-Stats videotapes of to study. I said how much I respected them and what an honor it was to be there. That it was a dream come true, because it truly was. "*But,*" I said, "all of that goes away when I'm competing, no matter who it is. It's no holds barred, get out of my way or get stepped on. Take no prisoners. I wasn't afraid of them because I was already so used to the men clobbering me in tournaments every week. I had to be confident. I don't see how you can win a match playing scared. So I just go for it."

Of course, in my naivety and lack of experience, I got to the next pro event and I found out that the top women were secretly passing around the magazine. The title read, in big bold letters, "Get Out of My Way or Get Stepped On" says Jeanette Lee. Great. Well, no wonder they hated me. The magazine had taken my quote out of context. That didn't help me at all.

I needed to make sure that never happened again. I needed more experience. I needed to know how to control an interview and say what I wanted to say instead of letting them lead me into what they wanted to hear. After that event, I went to the bookstore and bought over a dozen books on public relations, media relations, and marketing. Every time my back went out and I had to lay down, I was watching pool matches or reading a self-help book.

I got attention because the media wanted my attention, and I was happy to oblige. Of course I liked getting that attention, it seemed like a positive thing for both me and the sport, but being famous was never my goal.

As I rose to fame, I transcended cue sticks and eight balls, landing endorsements from companies like Bass Pro Shops, Ford, and Reebok, which had nothing to do with pool. I made corporate appearances for dozens of major companies, including Gatorade, Nordstrom, Lucas Oil, and Pepsi. My focus was on gaining the financial freedom to play pool as much as I wanted. I needed sponsors to make that happen. I worked on the red carpet at the *ESPYs* and lured a cult-like following.

My tournaments were aired on ESPN2 every weekend, and my face was splashed on magazine covers all over the world. In the 1990s and 2000s, I was the best-known pool player in the world, man or woman. I won Sportsperson of the Year in 1994 and 1999.

One poll during that time revealed that almost 70 percent of people in the United States knew the name Jeanette Lee and associated it with the sport of pocket billiards. I was among the most recognizable athletes in America, my name on lists alongside Michael Jordan, Peyton Manning, and Derek Jeter.

> "If she would walk through a casino like the Riviera on the Las Vegas Strip, within a minute or two, she couldn't move because there was a throng of people and they're descending on her. There was nothing like Jeanette Lee in the pool world."
> —Don Wardell, Lee's longtime physician and friend

I remember those walks through the casinos when it almost felt like those fans were suffocating me. It was intense. It was sometimes scary. But it was always rewarding. It was rewarding because it meant victory. I had risen to the top. I had overcome it all. I was the invincible Jeanette Lee.

Until I wasn't invincible anymore.

My toughest opponent came knocking at my door in 2021, wreaking havoc on my body and my soul. Stage 4 ovarian cancer.

My long black hair disappeared. I was tired, nauseous, and in pain. It was horrific. The cancer turned me into something I never wanted to be—a victim. It became almost impossible to imagine that I ever was indestructible, that I ever was The Black Widow.

Where was that woman, so strong, so confident, so ready to conquer the world? I knew she was still inside of me, somewhere. I would hear her pleading with me to fight, telling me I could beat this thing.

But The Black Widow seemed like a stranger to me now, and I was an outcast once again. And this time, I was an outcast fighting terminal cancer. Fighting for my life.

CHAPTER 2

WAS IT TIME FOR THE BLACK WIDOW TO DIE?

THE MONSTER CAME FOR ME IN THE DARK, as monsters usually do. It came for me suddenly, without warning, inside my bedroom in January 2021.

This monster was on an evil mission to destroy my life, shatter my soul, and then kill me. And this monster had a name, an ugly, well-known name: cancer.

The cancer had been there for a while, spreading throughout my body, invading my organs with clusters of tiny, abnormal, vicious cells.

But I didn't know that, not until that January night, when the monster finally appeared to me.

It was a cruel ending to what had been a magical Christmas. Just a few weeks earlier, my family had celebrated my favorite holiday. The revelry wasn't anything fancy, just Christmas in Tampa with plenty of good food, joyful laughter, gifts, and a lot of love.

It was just a normal holiday.

But normal is the only thing you want back, and normal seems absolutely incredible, after you hear the word "cancer."

I had just laid down in my bed that January night when my chest started pounding. It wasn't the kind of pounding that happens when your mind is racing as you try to fall asleep. It was more like my chest was being clenched.

I sat up in bed, gasping for air in the dark. I couldn't get a deep breath. I stood up in a panic, hoping the pressure would go away.

I had been through many panic attacks before. Maybe this was another one, and maybe I could get through it like I had all those other times before, those times when I felt like I was being suffocated.

I loved my fans. I adored my fans, but there were times, as the years passed, when their love for me became too much. I would have to hide inside a closet, or sneak into a bathroom stall and take deep breaths to calm myself down.

But deep breaths weren't working that night. I tried to rationalize the suffocation another way. Maybe I was just stressed about the world around me. The COVID-19 pandemic was at its peak, leaving death and destruction in its path. I was especially vulnerable to the virus, because I have two auto-immune diseases, which put me at very high risk. My daughters were having to be home-schooled, which was an awful struggle for them and for me. When the girls would go to see their dad, he and his new wife were having them watch videos on the dangers of the vaccine, the risks of wearing masks, and why they shouldn't allow themselves to be tested for COVID. Can you imagine how much that scared them and what a conflict that was when it came to my health? Our precious girls were being torn in opposite directions and I felt powerless to make it better.

My stress level was off the charts. The coronavirus was destroying my business as the sole owner of Tampa Bay APA, an amateur American Poolplayers Association franchise pool league. On top of that, I wasn't getting any more corporate appearances and lost almost all my sponsors—though, thankfully, APA kept me as their national spokesperson, and I still am.

Sleeping had not been easy for me during that time. I have always been a deep thinker, a person who wants everything to be okay, not just for me and my family, but for everyone around me. I've always liked helping people, taking care of people, serving people, and making them happy.

And I hated everything COVID was doing to America. If anything health-wise was heavy on my mind that night, it was the pandemic. My bank account was dwindling. I was a single mom to three preadolescent daughters. I was beyond stressed financially, and otherwise.

But as I paced my house that January night, I knew this feeling wasn't stress over the pandemic, and it wasn't a panic attack. It felt very different, and it scared me, so I prayed. *Please, God, let this pass.*

I woke up the next morning and the pressure in my chest was gone. I said a prayer of thanks and continued to work on my APA League with my office manager, Shylee.

But when I laid down in bed the next night, the weight came back, even heavier. It felt like a bowling ball was sitting on my chest. By the third night, I felt like I was drowning. I couldn't even lie down. I had to sleep with pillows propping me up.

The next morning, I packed my bags and my friend Julie took me to the hospital, where I tried to describe this feeling that I couldn't even explain in my own head. All I could tell the doctor was that when I laid down, it felt like I was choking. I assumed it was some type of respiratory infection.

For two straight days, two very long days, all they did was take test after test after test. Blood was drawn, spinal fluid was tested, and scans were done, but as I waited for the results, I never once thought of cancer. Never. Not one time did cancer cross my mind.

But then the monster reared its evil, ugly head.

My shortness of breath, doctors told me, was due to fluid that had built up between my lungs and chest.

That fluid was filled with cancerous cells that had started in either my ovaries or my uterus and had metastasized to my liver, abdomen, and peritoneum, the membrane that lines the cavity of the abdomen and covers the abdominal organs.

All I heard through a blur of medical terms was that I had cancer, and it was bad. It was the kind that had already spread, all the way up to my lungs.

But for some reason, as the doctor looked deep into my eyes and told me I was in the advanced stages of a disease that was causing cancer cells to swirl inside of me like a tornado, I didn't cry.

I didn't feel sadness, devastation, or even fear. All I felt was shock. All I felt was an unfathomable sense of disbelief. *Is this really happening to me? Cancer?* There was no space for any other emotion but shock. Not anger, not despair, and not feeling sorry for myself.

Why would I feel sorry for myself? Why would I succumb to the enemy? I never had before.

I was matter of fact with her, asking questions on how to cure the cancer.

I stood there, my head spinning, everything around me closing in on me, going dark.

The oncologist said I needed to start chemotherapy immediately. I wanted a second opinion. I will never forget the words my doctor said to me: "Ms. Lee, I'm sorry. You don't have time for a second opinion."

I never in my wildest imagination had expected to walk into that hospital and leave with a diagnosis of cancer. Thankfully, my cousin Jessica was able to get me an appointment with Dr. Jessica Stine, a surgeon who specialized in ovarian cancer. Three days later, in a room at Florida Cancer Specialists, she showed me scans of my body that lit up like a Christmas tree. All those bright, yellow spots were cancer, the doctor said. It was Stage 4. The doctor told me if I hadn't come in when I did, if I had kept ignoring my symptoms, I probably would have been dead within a month or two.

The odds were dire. I was 49 years old, and it was almost certain I wouldn't make it to my 50th birthday.

But for some reason, I didn't listen to the prognosis or the odds, not even when I was told that my cancer meant a less than 15 percent chance of surviving more than two years. What did odds really mean anyway? I had beaten the odds so many times before.

I was, after all, an outcast, a high school dropout and runaway teen who had conquered the world of pool. I had overcome racism, scoliosis, feelings of abandonment since my parents' divorce, and shame—and, more than that, a lifetime of surgeries and chronic pain from ankylosing spondylitis and fibromyalgia.

As that unwelcome opponent named cancer came demanding a match in January 2021, I was determined to overcome again.

> "Jeanette is the fiercest, most competitive player I've ever seen. She doesn't back down and she doesn't give up. And she took that fighting spirit from the pool table into her battle with cancer."
>
> —Don Wardell, Lee's longtime physician and friend

I walked into my house, hours after receiving my diagnosis, and I heard the laughter of my daughters, Cheyenne, Chloe, and Savannah. They sounded so happy and so carefree. They hadn't a worry in the world, other than typical kid stuff, teenage stuff, like clothes, friends, social media, and boys.

As I stood there listening to their laughter, an incredible wave of sadness rushed over me. How can I take this away from them? How can I take away their happiness?

I didn't want to tell my daughters I had cancer. I can't explain how desperately I did not want to tell them. I didn't want to take away their joy or their innocence. I was mortified that they would have to think about disease and death, that they would have to think about growing up without a mom.

But I knew the chemotherapy was going to change me. It was going to take away my long black hair, it was going to make me tired and weak, maybe worse. I knew I had to tell them.

Inside our Tampa home, with my daughters sitting in front of me on a couch in the living room, I had the toughest conversation I've ever had in my life. "Mommy has cancer," I said to them, trying not to cry. "But I'm going to fight this. There will be chemotherapy. My hair might fall out. It won't be easy. But we have to stay positive."

An eerie silence took over the room, as my daughters hung on to my every word. Then their silence turned to sounds of grief. I tried to reassure them. I told them repeatedly, "I'm going to fight this."

They kept saying, "Yes, I know, mommy." But they were crying, and that destroyed me. They were terrified.

I didn't tell them at the time, but I was terrified, too.

> "The terminal diagnosis, the treatments, the pain, that wasn't what worried Jeanette most. She made it clear from the very beginning that her biggest fear was leaving her daughters behind without a mom."
>
> —Tom George, Lee's longtime manager

As the days and weeks passed, the only thing in my mind was that I had to win this battle. Every time I thought about my girls growing up without me, it brought me to tears. I've had a great life, I love the Lord and I am saved. I'm going to a better place where my body won't hurt and I won't suffer all the cruelties of the world. I'm not afraid to die. But the idea of leaving my daughters without a mom... it was just unthinkable. *Unacceptable—not gonna happen.* That's what I kept telling myself while I pictured my girls graduating high school, falling in love, getting heartbroken, getting married, raising their kids, all without their mom to guide and support them.

That's when the unthinkable crept into my mind, a dark, terrifying thought: *Was it time for The Black Widow to die?*

And if I did die from this monster, this Stage 4 cancer, how would the world remember me?

Would the world remember me how I wanted to be remembered? As a kind person who loved her family and adored her fans? As an athlete who never turned down a request for an autograph, who mentored rookie players and sought to be the change I want to see in the world?

Would the world remember me as the underdog who prevailed? As a woman who overcame physical disabilities brought on by severe scoliosis, and who endured countless back surgeries, and unbearable pain?

Or would the world remember me as The Black Widow who wore sexy, black clothing, who was a fierce billiards powerhouse, who trampled opponents and became a media sensation?

Deep down, I knew the answer. Of course, they would remember me as The Black Widow.

But was I still even really The Black Widow? Or had cancer taken her away, too?

I had so many questions. How long did I have to live? Maybe a year or two? What did I need to do to prepare for my death? Had I done enough for my children? One of my daughters is autistic, agoraphobic, has ADHD, and severe anxiety and depression. What's to become of her? Who will give her the attention she needs? She is sweet and beautiful and strong, but she needs a lot of attention. Where would she live? What do I do with my business? Will I have to sell it? Had I done enough to impact the lives of others?

I felt myself reverting back to that young, insecure Korean American girl fighting to find her way. As the cancer ravaged my body, my heart, and my mind, it took me to places I hadn't been in decades.

It took me back to Brooklyn inside the towering apartment building where I grew up. It took me back to my childhood. It took me back to the beginnings of an unlikely billiards star, who never in a million years could have ever imagined she would one day be "The Black Widow."

It took me back to the complex journey of a girl born Jeanette Tak, whose biological father abandoned her.

CHAPTER 3

MY TWO DADS: FROM JEANETTE TAK TO JEANETTE LEE

NOBODY, NO ONE, and nothing in my life ever made me feel as special as my biological father, John Tak, made me feel when I was a little girl. Not my mother, not becoming the No. 1 pool player in the world, not my grandfather, not my husband, not my hall of fame induction, not my sister, and not the fans who swooned over me.

My biological dad transcended all of that. To me, he was absolutely perfect. He doted on me, laughed with me, hugged me, sang to me, comforted me, and made me feel like I was the most wonderful girl in the world, a girl named Jeanette Tak.

I was not born Jeanette Lee. Almost nobody, outside of my immediate family, knows that.

But in the East Flatbush neighborhood of Brooklyn, inside the Methodist Hospital of Brooklyn, I was born Jeanette Tak on July 9, 1971. My mother worked nearby at Kings County Hospital for decades as a nurse, until she retired at 65 years old.

My American name was Jeanette but, in Korea, the tradition was to have the elders name the child. My grandparents, neither of whom spoke English, gave me my Korean name, Jin-Hee, which together means bright, shining truth, or beautiful jewel.

My mother and my father brought Jeanette Tak home from Methodist Hospital that hot summer day to join my two-year-old sister, Doris, and a beautiful little family blossomed.

The first five years of my life were magical. I may have been tiny, but I have intense, vivid memories of my biological dad. John had so much passion, and he gave me so much love. He always made me feel like I was his favorite, and Doris probably thought she was his favorite, too. That's how special he made us both feel.

He would lift me and swing me around like an airplane. He would sing to us, read to us, play games with us, and play outside with us.

John would take us to Coney Island for cotton candy, the legendary wooden roller coaster, and the Ferris wheel, where we sat dangling above an enchanted world, inhaling the smell of Nathan's Famous hot dogs mingling with the aroma of fried dough dipped in cinnamon and sugar.

I'm not sure a girl could have asked for a better dad.

One day out of the blue, a devastating day that changed me forever, John was gone. He left when I was five years old, when he and my mother divorced.

I remember feeling an extreme sense of abandonment. I had no idea what had gone wrong. *What had I done wrong*? Was I not good enough? Was I not smart enough or pretty enough? I assumed he left because he didn't want us anymore, and I was crushed.

It crossed my mind that maybe John left because Doris and I fought too much, or because we made too much noise. It just didn't make any sense to me why he was gone.

John definitely was not perfect, but in my eyes, he was. He was a strong, comforting force, a kind, smiling, and loving man. I could not understand why my mother did not want to be married to him. Doris remembers things differently. She remembers my mother and John getting into heated arguments.

> "We knew, even being very little, that my mother and father were very mad at each other. You could hear the anger."
>
> —Doris Lee, Jeanette's sister

I don't remember my mom and John ever arguing. I don't remember their bickering, or their screaming, or them falling out of love. For me, it happened overnight. My biological father was gone for no reason at all, and I just wanted my daddy back.

I didn't see the faults that my mom saw in him.

John was an ambitious, but struggling, entrepreneur, always searching for the next way to make a fast buck. His day job was as the manager of Rainbow Supermarket, a New York City grocer that sold yogurt, canned goods, produce, and all sorts of other things.

But as John worked in the grocery industry, he would pour his money into riskier business ventures. Those ventures would, inevitably, fail. He would try another business, and that one would fail. He would invest in another business, and that one would fail, too.

Soon, there wasn't enough money for rent, groceries, or utilities. My parents' divorce and their arguments, I later found out, always revolved around money.

When John didn't have the cash he needed to pay off a loss or invest in his next crazy dream, he would take it from my mom. That was precious money to my mother, money she had earned toiling at her nursing job, money she wanted to use to make her family comfortable.

As my mom tried to fight John, he would tell her, "Your money is our money." John was not responsible in the way that my mother expected a husband to be.

My mother was the oldest of seven and John was the youngest of eight. Birth order can shape your personality in a big way. And in their case, it did.

John had wild dreams of making it big in America, but he could never make that happen. And my mom needed the money he spent on his wild dreams for rent. She was always worried about the here and now, feeding her children, buying school clothes, paying for doctor's appointments.

John was taking risks with our money, and that wasn't how my mom wanted to live. She didn't like risks. Those business ventures felt like gambling to her, and my mother was never a gambling woman. She believed in managing finances conservatively, working hard for the money to raise a family, and never blowing savings on some haphazard venture.

And that is why, I firmly believe to this day, my mother fell in love with Bo-Chun Lee, a frugal, stern man.

When my mom met Bo-Chun Lee, a few years after my parents divorced, he owned a fishery and would bring home imitation king crab sticks, the kind of crab sticks that you would find in a California sushi roll. My mom would sauté it, and that king crab literally melted in your mouth. It was divine and delicious.

But I wasn't so sure I loved the man who brought it home to us.

Bo-Chun Lee wasn't mean. He didn't mistreat us. He was just distant and gruff. He loved us in his own way. He would bring candy for Doris and me, and sea bass and shrimp for our mom.

When my mother started seeing Bo-Chun Lee, I could tell that she was happy. I could tell that she was relieved to have a companion, especially in the Korean culture where divorce is often looked at with shame. She wouldn't have to be a single mom raising two kids alone.

Bo-Chun Lee was divorced, too, with two sons and a daughter, who were already grown. He was 10 years older than my mother, and I knew that my mom liked Bo-Chun Lee. She had never had another man come to our apartment before. I knew they were seeing each other, but I didn't know how serious it had gotten.

Not until I went down to the lobby of our apartment building in January 1981, and bumped into my mom. She was all dressed up and looked gorgeous. I'd never seen her wear fake eyelashes before, and she was absolutely stunning. I realized at that moment that I definitely had the most beautiful mom in the whole neighborhood.

"Mom, you look so pretty." I could barely get the words out of my mouth before Bo-Chun Lee appeared, and he was dressed up, too.

They were dressed up because they had just gotten married. I was so hurt that they hadn't included me and Doris in their ceremony. Did our opinions not matter to them? Weren't we important enough to have been at their wedding? I was nine years old, and I felt so left out. I realized then that my mother was ashamed of us. She didn't want anyone to know that we existed.

Quickly after the wedding, my mom changed the name on my birth certificate from Jeanette Tak to Jeanette Lee, and she forced Doris and me to call Bo-Chun Lee "Daddy." I remember adamantly protesting. Tak was my last name, and it was the last thing I had of my real dad.

Bo-Chun Lee might have been my new stepfather but, in my mind, he would never be my dad. My mother would look in my eyes and say sternly, "He is your father now. You should call him 'Daddy.'" From then on, we called him "Daddy," and we still lovingly call him "Daddy" today. My mother told us that he would be a provider for us and that we had to share the same last name to be a family.

Daddy was Catholic, and he would get up each morning and pray with rosary beads, kneeling before a cross. He was now the head of our family and, if he was Catholic, we all had to become Catholic, too.

Before Daddy came into our lives, I had only been to Korean Presbyterian churches, and I have wonderful memories of that. It was the only time I was surrounded by Korean kids. I'm so thankful that my mom provided a place where, once a week, we fit in. No racism, no mean kids, just Korean kids that spoke English like us. We had an amazing youth pastor, who spoke Korean and English. This is where I learned about God and I built my faith in Jesus. It all made sense to me. And by God, I loved Jesus and I believed that the Holy Spirit was living inside me. I loved to worship Him and praise Him. I felt loved and protected by God. Especially since God loves his children so much! My mom sent me to Korean school every Saturday morning to learn to speak, read, and write Korean. I hated getting up early but I went because, again, I got to be around kids that looked just like me and shared the same Korean customs, traditions, and strict households, where we all had to study hard and practice piano or violin. It was nice to meet people with whom I had things in common.

My new Dad's Catholic church was very different than the funfillled Korean Presbyterian Church, which had an English-speaking youth ministry. It was very serious, very repetitive, and it was presented in all Korean, which I didn't understand. I never made a single friend at that church. Doris and I didn't enjoy going to mass in Korean. We couldn't get used to it, but we had no say in the matter.

My mother was ready for a fresh start, a new husband, and a new father figure for her two daughters. She liked the financial security Daddy brought. My mom respected that he was steady, and that she could count on him.

She knew when he was leaving, when he was coming back home, what he earned, and how he would contribute financially. It was the stability that my mom longed for, and Daddy gave her that stability. I will always be grateful to him for that.

Daddy wasn't rich. We weren't rich. We were barely middle class.

And yet, somehow, I never felt poor. It was all I knew, so I didn't feel deprived, at least not when it came to material things.

Emotionally, Daddy was never really there for me, and he certainly wasn't anything like my biological father. He never took me on Ferris wheel rides, or sang to me, or got down on the living room floor to play games with us. He never went to my school events or talked to me about life.

He was a different dad than I had known. He was a strict, religious, dependable, responsible husband and father. My biological father was hardworking, too. He just wasn't a great businessman, always changing his ideas, and taking risks on ventures that never flourished.

My mom couldn't depend on John Tak to help pay the bills, because he was always reinvesting his money in other business ideas. Bo-Chun Lee, on the other hand, would get up at 3:30 AM, eat breakfast, and leave by 4:30 AM to go to work. When he got home at 8:30 PM, he would eat dinner, watch TV, and be in bed by 10:00 PM. He would get up in the wee hours of the next morning and do it all over again.

Daddy believed a man's work was outside of the home. After the fishery, he owned a smoke shop in Manhattan across from the Empire State Building, and he worked even longer hours.

When he was at home, he sat in the living room and watched television—either the news or one Korean drama after another. His two chores were to vacuum the living room and take the garbage out each week. And if he saw dirty dishes in the sink, he would sometimes wash them, or pay me 50 cents to wash them. Those two quarters were like a million dollars to me.

I could get three Italian shaved ices with that money. I would run down to the shop and ask for a cup of my favorite flavor. Some days, it was coconut or cherry. Other days, it was blue raspberry or the rainbow cup. Those sweet towers of ice were a rare, indulgent treat, and I owed them to my new "dad."

But when I tried to tell Daddy thank you, he would grumble at me, with a smile. Don't get me wrong, Daddy was a nice guy, and a pretty likable guy if you could understand his English with his thick Korean accent and his gruff voice.

He was friendly if you talked to him, but we were never close to him. When he got home from work, he was always tired, and we would have to be quiet. My mother would tell us not to disturb him.

We were only to talk to Daddy if he talked to us first and, when he did, he would talk in short, terse sentences. "You good?" "Go help your mother." His voice was rough, husky, and loud.

My biological father's voice was soft, gentle, and loving. I missed him so much. I would think about all the little gifts he gave to us, the treats, the candies, and the tiny, yellow, stuffed cow that I named MooCow. I cherished that stuffed animal, and I carried her with me everywhere. It was the last thing I ever owned that reminded me of my father.

Daddy tried to be friendly, but it always seemed like he was a bit angry. He wasn't really angry, but we didn't know that. We didn't really know him.

If I was doing something wrong, Daddy would say, "What's the matter with you?" "What are you doing?" "Did you ask your mom?" And his favorite question: "Did you do your homework?" He and my mother were strict and intense about us being good students at school.

When he got home from work, he would call me over as he sat in his chair at the head of the table, drinking a beer, waiting for my mom to finish preparing his dinner. He would have me stand in front of him, and he would drill me on math questions. "What is 4 plus 4, plus 12, times 3, divided by 5?" "What is 81 divided by 9, plus 12, minus 17, times 3?"

I stood nervously, trying to answer his questions. I liked math, and the fact that he was challenging me. I didn't mind it, but I didn't love it, either. Especially when my mom would appear to serve Daddy his dinner, and he would forget all about me. I would walk away wondering why he had to be so serious, so hardworking, and so hard to get to know.

My biological father was the opposite of that. John Tak was an open book, he was funny, he was a risk taker, and he was a guy who didn't think life had to be some mundane routine made up of days that ran into one another. I am so much like my biological father.

I think that is why it hurt me so badly when he left us. One day, John was gone, and I didn't know why. After he left, my mother never spoke poorly about John in front of me. She never bashed him. She knew how much I missed him, and how much I loved him.

I don't think we ever talked about John after he left. I don't know why, but I never asked my mother why they divorced. Maybe it was because I was afraid to find out the truth, that it really was my fault that he was gone.

As I grew up, especially during the tough times, I would think about all the things I missed out on with my biological dad, the things he wasn't there for. I just knew he would have been different from my mother and stepdad.

I would have felt whole. I would have felt like I was good enough. I would have been part of something. Instead, I felt like a lost, little broken piece losing in the Game of Life. My parents were playing on one board, and I was on another board all by myself, lost and broken, and never measuring up to anyone around me.

My mom was loving in her own way, but she was not someone I could turn to. I never felt comfortable talking to her about my problems at school or the kids who were mean to me. I never felt like we really connected emotionally, on a deep level. I just remember that she was working all the time.

I remember her coming home so tired and trying to get sleep, but Doris and I would sometimes stay up talking and giggling. The walls were very thin in our little apartment, our bedrooms right next to one another. My mother would burst into our room and tell us to be quiet, because she really needed sleep.

I was sure if John had been there in that apartment, we would have had an intense connection. He would have wrapped his arms around me and comforted me about my problems at school with the other kids. He would have counseled me and told me everything was going to be okay. He probably would have walked me to school, so nobody would bother me or call me names.

I mourned the loss of my biological father, the man who had vanished with no trace.

When I was 19 years old, I got my chance to see John Tak again, to see if he was the man I remembered him to be. To find out if he was sorry for what he had done. To ask why he never wrote to me or called me.

My mom planned a trip to Korea to show me and Doris our heritage, and where we came from, though she had no intentions of reuniting us with John Tak. We visited Seoul, Busan, and Daegu. We went to the gravesites of our ancestors.

We visited our extended family, and stayed with girlfriends that my mother had gone to nursing school with when she lived in Germany. We visited my eldest uncle, my mom's only sibling who hadn't immigrated to America, and his wife and kids.

That trip really opened my eyes. I was a kid from Brooklyn, and while there were parts of Korea, such as Seoul, that reminded me of New York City, most of it was remote, rural, and rustic. In the fields, there were cows that looked like they had been starved. Their bones were protruding, and they had flies all over their faces. They smelled like death warmed over.

At most of the places we visited, there was no indoor plumbing, only outhouses, if we were lucky. In some areas, we had to squat to pee in the dirt. And you could forget about toilet paper. All of it was shocking to me. I always thought we were so poor, until I saw how most of these people were living in the country with no air conditioning in the heat of summer, and no furnaces in the dead of winter. It made me so thankful for the life that my mom and dad had provided.

It was a whole new world for me, a 19-year-old, up-and-coming pool star.

On that trip to Korea, I felt an overwhelming sense of being connected to my roots, my true heritage. I started thinking about my biological father and how wonderful it would be to see him again.

I went to my mom, nervously, one night, and I told her I wanted to find John Tak while we were in Korea. To my surprise, she didn't seem upset or alarmed at all. It was almost as if she had been ready for that question, just waiting for me to ask her that question all those years.

My mother quickly made a few phone calls and got in touch with John, who agreed to meet us. As his train arrived at the station, I stood waiting for him to step off, to see this man, my biological dad.

When he did, I ran into his arms and hugged him, like one of those Lifetime movies happening in slow motion. I felt this unreal wave of emotions—sadness, happiness, joy, and love. I felt like a giddy daddy's girl once again.

When John Tak wrapped his arms around me 16 years after he had left me, it was the first time in my life that I truly felt whole. I didn't realize, until that day at the train station in Korea, that there had been a big hole inside of me, a void haunting me all those years. I didn't realize it until John Tak filled it.

Mentally, emotionally, and spiritually, I was whole again. I remember thinking to myself, "Now I can handle anything. Everything's going to be good from this point on."

John and Doris and I toured Korea together, we ate meals together, and we went to temples together. We met John's daughters, Theresa and Rachel, two half-sisters we didn't know we had. They were nine and 11 years old at the time, exactly 10 years younger than Doris and me.

We went to visit their apartment, which was a humble space. There was a kitchen, a tiny living area, and a room the size of a closet, where my half-sisters slept next to a piano. My biological dad and his new wife slept in the living room, pulling out pads with blankets each night, and then rolling them up the next morning.

When I saw how they were living, I was sad, and I was shocked. I realized I was very lucky, and I was very blessed. Through the years, as I imagined what John was doing and where he was, I always assumed he was probably living in some lavish house, a rich happy man, thriving with a new family.

Instead, I saw a man who was much older and frail, who had a severe limp, moved slowly, seemed a bit sickly, and was studying acupuncture. Honestly, I could have spent that whole summer just staring at his face, taking it in, and never forgetting what he looked like.

Doris was glad to see John, too, but she was far less trusting of him. She, after all, had memories of the fights between my mother and John that I didn't remember. She loved him just as much as I did, but she was more loyal to my mom because she knew what our mother had gone through.

On that trip to Korea, I found out John had been struggling for 16 years to make ends meet. On that trip, I learned that after he left us, when I was five years old, he had tried to stay in touch. Through the years, John had tried to call and write to me and Doris, but my mom had told him to stay away. She would tell him, "Just let them grow up. I'm remarried, and Bo-Chun Lee is their dad. Let us be a family."

I didn't know any of that, not until I was 21, standing in my biological father's home in Korea. Now I could finally forgive John. It wasn't his fault. He really did care about us. He had tried to stay in touch.

And that's what he told me again, all those years later. He wanted to stay in touch with me, and he wanted to build a relationship. I was absolutely elated.

As I left Korea, I had newfound hope that John would be part of my life. As soon as I got back to New York, I wrote to him and his family, and they wrote me back. I sent another letter, and they wrote me back again. It was wonderful getting to be a part of my biological dad's life again and to have two little sisters.

But after the fifth letter, John Tak did it again. He abandoned me. He didn't write back. He stopped all contact. I still tried to call and write, still longing for his love, but I got no response. Nothing. Doris tried to write to him, too. Nothing. He just stopped all communication with us.

For the second time in my life, I felt extremely abandoned. I thought to myself, "How much does a stamp cost? How tough is it to send a letter?" That's when I closed my heart to John Tak and said, "Okay, that was your second chance. Now we're done. We are done."

I became bitter. And I poured my heart and soul into pool, mostly because I loved it, but partly because it was an escape from feeling unwanted by my biological father. It was painful to realize that John would never walk me down the aisle, never teach me how to drive or go to a school play or be there when a boyfriend broke my heart.

I would never be the daughter I wanted to be, because I was missing the father who I always wanted to really love me.

A couple of years after John Tak deserted me for the second time, I became the No. 1 women's pool player in the world. I'd become a sports superstar, and I was living in Long Beach with my new husband, a fellow star pool player, George Breedlove. And that's when I got the call from my Aunt Dorothy that John had moved to San Francisco and wanted to see me.

My head was spinning. *Are you kidding? Really? No way. I did not want to see John Tak.* But my father's family kept calling me. They would say, "Don't you want to see him? He's your father."

I told them that I didn't believe a father was someone who abandoned their children. I told my family bluntly: "My father is in New York."

By that time, I had finally realized and accepted that Daddy was the only father I had really ever had in my life. He may not have been there for me emotionally, but he always made sure I had what I needed, he was someone my mom could count on, and he truly loved my mother.

I loved and respected Daddy greatly for that. I appreciated him for filling the role my mom wanted for us. While he and I didn't really have deep conversations, he would always tell me how much he prayed for us. He still does to this day.

But my biological father's family would not stop calling me, begging me to see John Tak, and that made me angry. I didn't get it. Why was it so important to them that I see him now, just because he had moved to San Francisco?

Where were they when he was abandoning me and Doris? Why hadn't they called John all those years ago and told him, "You have daughters in New York City. Why don't you see them?" I didn't know how to tell them that I didn't want to risk having my heart broken for the third time.

"The next time one of you calls me, bugging me to go see John Tak, it'll be the last time I speak to you," I told my father's family. "If you cannot respect me as an adult and my feelings, then you are not welcome to call me again." I know they did it out of love but I needed a break. They were always so kind to me but I was too upset.

Their calls finally stopped, and a little time passed. But that time didn't take away the hurt and resentment I felt that John Tak was trying to come back into my life. I thought I had buried all that pain, but I found myself crying a lot. I poured my heart out to my new husband, George Breedlove, lamenting the biological father who had abandoned me twice.

George disagreed with my resistance to reunite with John Tak, and he eventually took it into his own hands.

"Let's go for a drive," George said to me one day. We were living in L.A. at the time. As I sat in the passenger seat on that drive, I spilled my guts out, talking about all the things I wished my father would have given me, done with me, and how much he had hurt me.

We drove for hours, and I talked for hours about my father. And then George stopped the car. "Let's go," he said to me.

Where? Where were we? "Where are we going?" I asked George. It was a mixture of anger and confusion when I found out where we were. George had driven me to San Francisco, to my biological father's home.

"You need to see him," George said to me, as he looked deep into my eyes. I fought it. I screamed at George. "Where was he the last five years? Where was he my entire life?"

George was level-headed and insistent, and he said, "I don't want you to see him for him. I want you to see him for you, so that you can have closure."

I reluctantly agreed to meet with John Tak that day, fuming inside. I was sure that he would give me some lame excuse for his lack of contact, and I was worried about how I would react. I knew I could not handle that rejection again.

George told me to go in with an open mind and just listen to what John had to say, and so I did. I was nervous, emotional, and, deep down, absolutely terrified.

I met my biological dad for his third chance at a restaurant, an Asian all-you-can-eat buffet. He walked up to me and said, "Hello, hi, this is John." He didn't say, "This is your father." I liked that. And when he talked, he didn't make excuses.

All John said to me that day was that he was so happy to see me and that he was so happy about my success. He was very gentle, very calm, very tired, and, in many ways, looked very broken. But could I trust this third incarnation of John Tak?

The first time I reunited with him, I was a 19-year-old nobody, a fledgling pool player. But now, I was the No. 1 women's billiards player in the world. I was on magazine covers, on popular talk shows, in newspapers, and playing championship matches on ESPN2.

In the back of my mind, I thought, "Oh, now John wants to be in my life? Isn't that convenient?"

But as quickly as those thoughts crept into my mind, they dissipated. John didn't ask me for anything that day, and he never did. Deep down, I knew my biological father wanted to see me because he loved me, and he wanted to make things right between us.

We didn't discuss what happened that day, why he had suddenly stopped writing to Doris and me, and John made no excuses. To my surprise, I ended up being relieved and happy to have reunited with my father and his family.

This time, John Tak didn't leave me. We stayed in touch. He and his family came to visit us in L.A., and when we moved to Indiana, Rosy asked to live with George and me for her four years of high school. I was elated and so happy to have that time with her.

I always wished I'd had that time with John, and Rosy was an extension of him. She and I would visit our father and talk to him on the phone.

Throughout the years, John and I made a few wonderful memories. But this wasn't some fairy tale ending to a father-daughter relationship. In my mind, it was too little too late. I was never going to get what I had missed, all those years growing up without him. My heart was hardened to John because of all the abandonment.

But as the years passed and John became older and frailer, my heart began to soften, and then it began to melt, and then forgiveness set in. John hadn't come back in my life because I was a famous pool player. He just wanted to be part of my life. In the end, it only mattered that I still loved him, and that I knew he loved me back.

But in 2006, John Tak left me again, for the final time. "I think dad is really sick," Rosy called to tell me. I booked plane tickets, and we flew to be with John at the hospital. Doctors told us that his body was shutting down, that he couldn't breathe on his own.

I stood there looking at John Tak lying in that hospital bed, so weak, so worn out. I told him that I loved him, and that I forgave him. I told him how wonderful it had been to be his daughter when I was a little girl, and how he had made me feel so special.

I desperately wanted him to hear, in those final hours of his life, that he had made me feel like the most wonderful daughter in the world. Even though he was sleeping, not able to breathe on his own, I believe that John heard my words. I am choosing to believe he heard my words.

Minutes later, as I lay next to him in his bed, holding John Tak in my arms, he took his last breath.

I left the hospital that night with one father left in my life. Bo-Chun Lee was, in truth, the only father I ever really had. He had been with me since I was nine years old, supporting me in the only way he knew how.

Throughout my life, I had two fathers. Some would say that was a blessing, and it was. But it was also complicated. My childhood, after all, was not filled with the stuff superstar pool players' dreams are made of.

CHAPTER 4

FADING MEMORIES OF A WONDERFUL AND WOEFUL CHILDHOOD

MUCH OF MY EARLY CHILDHOOD has become one big, hazy blur—fading memories stolen by the years that have passed, by the pain, the trauma, the chemotherapy, the cancer, and who knows what else.

Since my Stage 4 cancer diagnosis, I often feel like my brain is mush. That's the best way I can describe it. Sometimes I will be talking and mid-sentence I can't remember what I was saying. Sometimes it feels like entire years of my life have vanished. And then, without warning, they'll pop up again.

I still remember tidbits of my childhood growing up as a scrawny Korean American girl who was part shy, part happy, part sad, and part rebel. There are wonderful memories and there are terrible memories, and there are memories I swear happened, yet my family swears they didn't.

But for some reason, I can still remember every single detail of that towering 16-story apartment building in New York, in the East Flatbush neighborhood of Crown Heights, Brooklyn, where I grew up.

There were double glass doors at the entrance to that building at 636 Brooklyn Ave., which in my eyes seemed as tall as the Empire State Building, where a doorman sat behind a counter on the right.

He was part security guard, especially when night would fall, asking the people who tried to walk inside who they were, what apartment they lived in, and, if he could confirm they were residents, ushering them in.

During the day, the doors to the building were usually open, but the doorman was more greeter than guard. He knew our names, said hello as we walked in, and sometimes he would let Doris and I go behind the counter with him, which made us feel really important.

Just inside the building were 160 mailboxes for each of the 160 apartments. They looked like tiny lockers stacked side by side, one on top of the other. We would open our mailbox and find letters from relatives in Korea, bills, and all sorts of fliers and ads for restaurants, grocery stores, and entertainment in New York City.

Beyond the mailboxes was the lobby of our building. It was a sparse, functional lobby. There weren't posh couches or works of art on the walls, like fancy apartment buildings had. Our lobby was nothing more than a place to walk through to get to the elevator, or the door that opened to the staircase, which went up 16 flights.

All throughout the building, the paint on the walls was dingy, kind of a beige color. It was obvious it was supposed to be white, but it hadn't been cleaned in years.

Each floor of the building was one big rectangle with laminated floors, or maybe tile squares, that were dark brown and dotted with tiny specks of lighter brown. To this day, I can still smell exactly what that building smelled like. Kind of dank, kind of musty, and filled with the aroma of cigarettes, roach spray, and fried food.

My family lived in apartment 12C. When you got off the elevator on the 12th floor and turned left, there was apartment 12A, then 12B, and then 12C. If you made your way around the rectangle back to the elevator, you would end up at 12J.

Inside our apartment was a small kitchen, a modest living room, three bedrooms, a bathroom, and a row of windows that looked out onto Brooklyn Avenue and Wingate Park. Even as a young girl, I remember always wanting to get outside of that apartment building.

There was a massive steel door in the lobby that led to the backyard, which had a big statue of a turtle, and one basketball hoop with no net. There was no swing set, seesaw, or merry-go-round. But Doris and I and the other children who lived in the building would run around in the backyard, playing tag and concocting silly games.

> "We were really active, riding our bikes, playing games, and playing tag. We had cuts and bruises and mosquito bites all over our arms and legs. We had bandages on all the time from falling. We were just always going, going, going."
>
> —Doris Lee, Jeanette's sister

No matter what we were playing, I was always really competitive. I always wanted to destroy the boys. We would play cards, a game called Spit. We would play basketball. We would throw the football and, sometimes, we would just sit in the grass as darkness fell and talk—until our mom forced us to come inside.

That apartment building may have been a modest place to call home. It may not have been a luxurious high-rise, but it was the American dream for my mother, Sonja.

In 1968, in her late twenties, my mother had immigrated to the United States from Korea with big dreams, looking for better opportunities and a better life.

In the 1960s, the U.S. had a demand for nurses and medical professionals, and my mom was part of a wave of nurses—including my mom's classmates from nursing school—that went from Korea to Germany, and then from Germany to the U.S. Many other Koreans also immigrated to the U.S. in those years in search of work.

My mother had been born in Korea in 1940, when it was one undivided country. She was raised in southern Korea, the oldest of seven siblings, and she graduated top of her class in high school. My mother should have gotten to go to college. She had the grades, and she definitely had the smarts.

But her family only had enough money to send one child to college. And that money went not to my mother, but to her younger brother, my grandparents' oldest son.

Still, my mother forged ahead and, after graduating nursing school, went to work as a nurse in Germany. She married John Tak and moved to Brooklyn. By the mid-1970s, when I was a toddler, my mother's parents and all but one of her seven siblings, immigrated to the United States and moved into that apartment building with us.

My memories from that time may be fading, but not all of them have vanished. I remember some wonderful things, and I remember some not so wonderful things.

> "I don't know why, but for some reason Jeanette has very dark memories from our childhood. I don't have those. But she does."
>
> —Doris Lee, Jeanette's sister

I remember battling racism, and that was hard for me. We lived in a neighborhood that was filled with mostly Black families, a few White families, and no Asian families. I remember being taunted because I was Asian.

Doris doesn't remember it being so terrible. She says the racist comments happened only on occasion. To me, it felt like those comments came every single day, kids making fun of the shape of my eyes, my skinny body, and my heritage.

I felt like an entire neighborhood was against one Korean family—my family. I was young. I felt hated, and I didn't understand why. And, as I've said, I didn't understand why my father left either, and I blamed myself for him leaving, always wondering what I had done wrong.

With John Tak gone from our lives, my mom became a single mother, raising two girls on her own. Luckily, she had the means to provide for us financially, but that came with a sacrifice. We didn't get to spend much time with my mother.

She was a registered nurse at Kings County Hospital and she worked long, excruciating hours. I don't remember her being around.

I didn't have a close relationship with my mother growing up. I loved her, and she gave me unconditional love, but she didn't toss me in the air or play games with me.

She just worked very hard. She worked two or three jobs. My mother would finish her regular shift as a nurse at the hospital, then pick up extra shifts. When she wasn't at the hospital, she would sell jewelry on the side.

When I was nine years old, my mother married Bo-Chun Lee, who I consider my dad, and he worked even longer hours than she did. He was even more distant than she was, and he focused on what he believed was the only thing a man should be focusing on, providing for his family.

It wasn't unusual for Doris and me to be left home alone, mostly to fend for ourselves, especially because we had our grandparents and aunts and uncles in the building, living in apartments 10C, 9J, 15B, and 4C.

Whenever we needed anything, Doris and I would just go to a family member, for a homecooked meal, for help with homework, for a haircut, or for something more dire, like the day I cut off the tip of my finger trying to remove the stalk from a sugar cane.

Sugar canes were a treat in Southeast Asia, a treat my mom liked to give us, but to eat them the tough skin had to be removed. Usually, my mom would cut the sugar canes and let Doris and I chew them, sucking out all the juice and sugar. Those sugar canes were the best treat in the world.

But one day, I wanted a sugar cane and my mom wasn't home. So I took a butcher's knife, went for the stalk and, suddenly, there was blood everywhere. I had sliced off the tip of my finger.

I grabbed a wad of napkins or, maybe it was a dishcloth, ran out of my apartment, and started knocking on the doors of every family member in the building. I was holding a piece of my dismantled finger and shrieking, "Oh no! Oh no, no, no! My finger is gone!"

Finally, I found my Aunt Ruth, who was at home, who happened to be a nurse. She calmed me down, sterilized my wound, and she secured my finger back together with Steri-Strip medical tape.

I went to school the next day with my battle scar and I bragged to classmates, who begged to see my gory injury. As the days followed, I started peeling off the medical tape so my friends could see the insides of my finger, the gooey flesh. They oohed and ahhed over what I had been through, and I felt kind of important.

But each time I pulled off the tape, my finger got worse. There was no way it could heal.

My mom was furious when she found out what I was doing. She said very sternly, "Jeanette, stop doing that. You have to let your finger heal."

Growing up, my mother was the disciplinarian. Neither of my fathers played that role, even a little bit. If Doris or I acted up, my mother would be the one who spanked us. She was the one who told us to stop fighting. She was the one who set rules for bathing, chores, and bedtime.

But she also tried to do wonderful things for us, little things that made us feel loved. My mother made delicious food for us. She bought a deep fryer, a newfangled cooking device in the 1970s, and would make this amazing fried chicken.

She would make peanut butter and honey sandwiches. In the hot days of summer, she would concoct *sikhye*, an incredible, sweet rice beverage, traditionally served as a dessert drink.

My mom always tried to do things that made us feel special. She would take us to Sears for family portraits. She would take us to the circus. She would take us to the beach.

After the divorce, my mother saved up enough money to take me, Doris, and our grandmother to Disney World in Florida with her best friend, who had daughters our age. That trip was magical.

On my birthdays, I always got my very own bucket of Kentucky Fried Chicken. That was my favorite food in the world. I loved the original recipe, the only version the restaurant offered at the time, long before the crispy and extra crispy varieties came on the menu.

I loved the drumsticks the best, and I loved mixing the mashed potatoes with the coleslaw. I thought that was the most delectable combination of food I had ever tasted.

My dad eventually sold the fish store and bought a smoke shop across the street from the Empire State Building that sold cigarettes, cigars, magazines, lottery tickets, and candy. The first time I walked into the tiny shop and saw all that candy, I was mesmerized.

There, spread out in front of me in his shop, was bubble gum, Pop Rocks, Laffy Taffy, licorice sticks, lollipops, every color of Tic Tacs you can imagine, and every variety of chocolate bars made. Snickers, Milky Ways, Twix, 100 Grands, and peanut butter cups.

Growing up, I don't remember getting to have play dates. I never had any friends come to my apartment and I wasn't allowed to go to any of my friends' apartments. We would just meet in the backyard to play. I didn't know if that was normal. I didn't have anything to compare it to. That was just the way things were.

At home, I always got a lot of praise, a lot of encouragement from my mother. But there were also strict rules. We were discouraged from watching TV. After we took a shower or bath, we had to get down on our hands and knees and scrub the whole tub. We had to get our homework done first, and if Mom was home we had to practice the piano, usually during the same time that I knew my friends were outside playing. I always resented my mom for that and I swore to myself that I would never play the piano again when I became independent.

I had to go to Korean School every Saturday morning with my cousins and clean our room every weekend. We couldn't make much of a mess, after all, because we really didn't have much. We certainly weren't spoiled. I do remember being obsessed with Michael Jackson. I had one of his posters on my wall and several Michael Jackson tin pins that I wore on my clothes and put on my bags.

At Christmas, Doris and I got a few small gifts with a tag from Santa in my mom's handwriting. It wasn't like the Christmases we saw on TV where dozens of expensive gifts, wrapped with ribbons and bows, were found underneath a glistening, seven-foot tree.

I was okay with that. I was just fine with that. I don't want to insinuate that my childhood was awful. It wasn't awful. There were plenty of happy memories, playing in the backyard or playing games with my sister and cousin Esther. I felt very loved by my mom, my grandparents, and all my aunts and uncles and cousins who lived in our apartment building.

And yet, for some reason, I started to rebel at a very early age. I was only nine years old, a tiny fourth grader, when I smoked my first cigarette. I remember really liking that feeling of doing something bad.

My *harabeoji* (Korean for "grandfather"), Hee Soo Kim, was the only person in all our generations to smoke cigarettes (that is, until I secretly followed after him). Because he was the patriarch of the family, he was allowed to smoke wherever he wanted, including inside our little apartment.

Sometimes he would forget his cigarettes at our place, and I would wait until I was alone in the house, stick my head out the window, and smoke a cigarette whenever I felt like being bad. Later, when Daddy bought the smoke shop in Manhattan, I'd take any opportunity I could to help out on the weekends so I could eat candy and steal packs of cigarettes. As I got older and bolder, I'd sometimes steal an entire carton.

I never planned to be a smoker. As a little girl, I had always hated smoking, the idea of inhaling toxins into your body and the awful, suffocating smell that permeated the room. I remember begging my grandfather to throw away his poisonous sticks and quit his deadly habit.

At that time, I was obsessed with the cartoon series *The Smurfs*, which featured lovable, little blue creatures. I would craft *Smurfs* posters and signs that said, "No smoking," or "I hate smoking," and I would hang them on the walls or bedroom doors inside my grandparents' apartment.

I may have hated his smoking, but I loved my grandfather. I loved my grandmother too. They often had to watch us when we were too young to be on our own. We would play traditional Korean board games, like Omok and Baduk. He also spoke a little English, whereas my grandmother really didn't, which made me feel so close to him.

In typical Korean households, the children played with the children. It wasn't common for adults to sit and play with the kids. The adults would watch TV, read the Bible, or talk to other adults. But my grandfather was cool. He had been a well-known soccer champion who traveled throughout Korea and, eventually, wrote a best-selling autobiography.

As a little girl, all I wanted was to be perfect in my grandfather's eyes.

> "Jeanette wanted to please. She was a child who liked to please you, and she was very innocent and sweet."
>
> —Doris Lee, Jeanette's sister

But by the time I was nine, sneaking to smoke cigarettes, those days of trying to please people were dissipating.

I know I didn't feel close to my mom or my dad at the time, and I know I didn't like the ritualistic rules my mom had in place. All I knew was that I felt hated by my sister and angry at my mom for some reason, and I just wanted to run away.

I ran away a few times when I was around 11, but I always came back. After all, where would I go? I had never been to any friend's house. But when my mom pulled me out of a horrid middle school to go to a private school in Manhattan, I made a few friends. It was a primarily White school but, for whatever reason, there was less racism. I would crash on couches at the homes of whatever classmates' parents would take me in. I was trying to find acceptance. Usually, it wasn't acceptance that I found. It was more pity.

My mom had no idea where I was for weeks at a time, and I didn't care that my parents were back home frantic and extremely worried. I feel awful about that now. But at the time I didn't feel awful at all.

After couch-hopping from house to house, I finally found a permanent way to be away from home. To this day, I can't remember exactly how it happened, but I was a young teen when my science teacher, Ernie, and his wife took me in.

They allowed me to live with them on two conditions. First, I had to call my mother and let her know I was okay, that I was safe. I had to give her the phone number to their home where she could reach me any time.

Second, I had to earn my keep. My teacher had 12 pet birds. It was my responsibility to feed them, clean their cages, and scrub away the bird poop. That gave me my first taste of responsibility, and that was good for me.

But it wasn't enough to settle this chaotic time. Eventually, I went back home. But things weren't better at first. My mom continued to try to reel me in, gain control over her rebelling daughter, but she was the last person I wanted to be around. It's not her fault but I just felt like a disappointment all the time, even though she never treated me as such. We loved each other so deeply, but our worlds were too different and I didn't believe she would ever understand me.

But when I moved back home, she allowed me to decorate my bedroom my way. I painted my room metallic black and bought a black bedside lamp. For my 13th birthday, she got me a pretty Korean black ashtray with cherry blossoms and a beautiful white crane in mother of pearl. It sounds crazy but I think she wanted me to feel as though she was accepting me—and it worked. I was so surprised but touched at the gift, as though she was showing that she was trying to compromise, meeting me halfway, instead of me constantly feeling like I had to live up to something. I appreciated it.

This was just the beginning of my downward spiral, which only intensified a year later when scoliosis came for me and turned my life upside down.

CHAPTER 5

BECOMING A MONSTER

THE WICKED CURVE of my spine was discovered on a hot, summer afternoon at Long Beach Island, where the sun was glistening, the sand was white, and a perfect breeze blew on our faces. My mom had taken the day off work to spend a glorious day at the beach with us, which was wonderful, and a bit shocking at the same time.

My mom never missed work unless it was for a very good, logical reason, like an important appointment or a funeral. Frivolities weren't really part of our lives but, on occasion, my mom would make time for them. And on this day, she had taken Doris and me to the ocean.

As I took off my shirt that day at the beach, revealing my skinny, 12-year-old body in a swimsuit, that's when my mom saw it. She saw the curve in my back.

I had just started running toward the water when I heard her scream, "Come back here, Jeanette. Come back here."

The ocean would have to wait for a new insecurity to wash over my body.

My mom stood in the sand, and she pulled me close to her. She put her fingers on my back, and she ran them up and down my spine.

I stood there and watched Doris splashing in the waves, as my mom told me to bend over and stand up. Bend over again. Stand up again.

"Walk in front of me," she said sternly. "Now, stand still." As my mom looked at my thin body from behind with bones protruding, she knew. She was a nurse, after all.

My mom didn't say the word "scoliosis" to me that day. That awful word would come later from doctors, who were stunned that I was even able to function with a spine as crooked as mine.

"Your back," my mom said to me, trying not to sound panicked, as we stood on the beach. "It doesn't seem right."

My mom hadn't seen me naked in years. By the time Doris and I were seven or eight years old, we bathed ourselves. I had no idea how long the curve had been there. But when my mom saw the bend in my spine that day, she was terrified.

> "Other than this, we never had any surgery or big disease, so it was a pretty big deal. My mom was very, very worried. There was something wrong with her daughter."
>
> —Doris Lee, Jeanette's sister

Our glorious beach visit turned gloomy. I'm not sure if I even got to splash in the ocean that day. I just remember packing up our towels and going home, where my mom quickly started calling doctor's offices for appointments.

As I listened to her frantic voice from my bedroom, I still didn't understand why it was such a big deal that I had a bend in my back. There was no internet in the 1980s. Google didn't exist. There was no way for a 12-year-old girl to quickly search what curvature of the spine meant.

I had no idea when I walked into that doctor's appointment that I had anything to be too worried about. I didn't feel nervous. I went through endless X-rays and tests, and then I sat with my mom and listened as the doctor said to me, "You have severe scoliosis."

I wasn't startled by that. The word scoliosis meant nothing to me.

The doctor showed us several X-rays of my back and, in every single one, my spine looked just like the letter "S." A person's spine is supposed to be straight, more like a lowercase "L." The doctor droned on with all sorts of incomprehensible medical terms, and a blur of numbers.

A normal spine might have a curvature of zero to 10 degrees, he said. But my spine was 58 degrees and 56 degrees of crooked, a double curve. Some people with scoliosis just have a C-shaped curve, meaning one bend. But both the top and bottom of my spine were curved, and both were considered on the very severe end of severe scoliosis.

If something wasn't done, doctors told us, the curves would only get worse, and they would be debilitating. This scoliosis had to be "nipped in the bud," they said.

I had no idea what that meant until a surgeon performed an operation to try to nip my scoliosis in the bud and I woke up from anesthesia with the most unbearable, excruciating pain I had ever felt. It literally permeated my body.

Inside the operating room, the surgeons had dismantled my spine, broken it open, and implanted two 18-inch Harrington rods. Those shiny, stainless-steel rods, foreign matter to a human body, were lined up against my spinal column with dozens of wire threads clipping the rods to my vertebrae.

When the surgery was over, the doctors weren't pleased. My spine was such a mess that, in the operating room, they determined there was no way they could straighten my back the way they wanted to. They told my mother they did the best they could.

The surgery improved the curvature of my spine to 28 degrees, still considered moderate scoliosis. But 28 was better than 56 or 58, doctors said, and I believed them—until 28 degrees was traumatic, and horrific, and all I wanted to do was die.

The trauma my body went through from that surgery caused me to grow three and a half inches, literally, overnight. The day after surgery, I was nearly four inches taller. My spine had been forced to stretch out, to do things that it didn't want to do, and my body fought back with a vengeance.

I would wake up in my hospital bed in agony, so drugged that I couldn't speak. I desperately wanted to scream out, to tell the doctors and my mom how much pain I was in. I remember tears streaming down my face as I looked into my mother's eyes, screaming on the inside, "Mom, help. This hurts too much."

But I couldn't get my mouth to move or the words to come out. I felt like I was dying from the pain, but nobody knew. I suffered in silence. Pain medicine back then was not like it is today. Rather than easing the pain, it just made me numb and sluggish. I was completely doped up and yet I still felt so much pain.

When I was sent home to recover, the misery didn't end. My mom would sit next to me, hold my hand, and she would pray. As she pleaded with God to take away my suffering and heal me, I laid in that bed and thought, "What the hell is this? What the hell is going on?"

I wasn't told before the surgery how awful the aftermath would be, and I wasn't told that the pain from that surgery was only the beginning of the trials that would follow me for the rest of my life. In the early 1980s it wasn't like it is today, where parents are offered support groups and resources.

As I recovered, I had a giant, white cast that covered my entire torso and extended over both shoulders. It was hot, itchy, and really heavy. I had to wear that for almost four months.

After lying immobile in bed for so long, atrophy set into my legs. They were so weak, I couldn't walk on my own. No one had told me this operation would force me to learn how to walk again.

I felt like a stumbling, wobbly scarecrow, trying to use the walker the doctors gave me. I would try to get my balance, and I would try to feel my feet underneath me, but sometimes I couldn't feel my feet at all.

Without the walker, I was like a toddler stumbling my way from the couch to the table, grasping for anything I could hold on to. I willed my mind to focus and my feet to move. I practiced from morning until night, day after day, looking forward to the day when this awful cast would come off.

I thought I would be free after the cast was removed. I thought I would feel normal. I was wrong.

The doctors had to make sure the surgery stuck, to make sure my spine stayed in the position they wanted it to be in, to protect the instrumentation they had inserted into my body. And that meant I had to wear a giant, clunky, hard-plastic, yellow brace. No one had warned me about the brace before my surgery.

I wasn't normal. I was a monster. With nowhere to hide.

Before school each day, my mom would place one piece of the plastic brace on the front of my body, and she would place the other piece of the brace on my back. She would take big Velcro straps across metal rings and secure the two braces tightly together.

The braces chafed against my collarbone at the top of my body and against my pelvis at the bottom, where the braces ended.

There were no clothes I owned that could cover the bulky brace, which was a pinkish, light beige that didn't match the color of my skin. I always had to wear men's tank tops to go under and up around the brace to keep raw blisters from forming. My mom would take the straps of the tank top and pull them tightly on my neck and pin them together.

I had to wear baggy men's jogging pants that would fit around the brace on my waist, and I had to wear long-sleeved, baggy shirts to try to hide the bulk.

In my mind, I looked like Frankenstein.

When I went to the restroom, I had to hoist the bottom of the brace up with one hand as I used the other hand to pull down my pants and underwear. I had to sit on the toilet, holding the brace up as I went to the bathroom. It was a shameful position to be in. That brace was pure evil.

> "I remember teasing her and knocking on the brace because it was plastic and she really hated that, because then people would be aware of it. She just wanted to go back to normal as soon as possible."
>
> —Doris Lee, Jeanette's sister

I was, after all, a middle school girl with insecurities raging, along with my hormones. I was a girl who had crushes on cute guys. Deep down, I knew there was no way those cute guys would ever look my way. I knew they would never see me as anything other than a weird girl with a brace.

And then there were all the girls in school who had their cool cliques made up of gorgeous cheerleaders and athletes and smart student body leaders. I desperately wanted to be friends with those girls, any of those girls, but they saw me as nothing more than a misfit, a loser who wore a brace.

Imagine being in middle school, when kids are at their meanest, and having to go through that torture.

To be honest, I hated being alive.

I didn't fit in anywhere. I felt like an ugly unwanted moth, hoping to be noticed, to be liked, trying to find a place to land and be accepted. To be honest, I still feel like that, more often than I would like. I have never found a way to fit in, except when I'm playing pool, except when I'm recognized as "The Black Widow." I had to learn to go through life struggling to find a way to be okay with being different.

When I stopped trying to fit in, I was able to start focusing on what I really wanted out of my life.

I have never been the woman with a huge circle of close friends who all hang out together, going to movies and restaurants and plays, or going on adventurous, girls-only weekend trips.

But through the years, I have made a lot of friends who I love, respect, and trust. They are friends I met through my pool travels, and the places I've lived, from the East to the West Coast, and back again. I feel so thankful for those friends.

When I was 13 and battling scoliosis, I didn't have any friends and depression set in like a dark cloud hovering above me. In the 1980s, people didn't talk about mental health and, when they did, it was usually about "crazy people" and stigmas, not about regular people who suffered from anxiety or depression.

As a young teenage girl wearing a brace, all I knew was that I felt sad, worthless, and ugly. To get through those feelings, I started to develop dangerous habits.

I would go to my grandfather's apartment, sneak out his cigarettes, and race back to my apartment. My mom and dad were always working, which gave me plenty of time to light up. At first, I would put my face out the window as I smoked to hide the smell, but the clouds still seeped into the room.

I soon came up with a different, dangerous plan. I would hang my entire body out the window of apartment 12C. I would sit on the windowsill with one leg out, and one leg in, most of my body more on the outside than on the inside.

If the people on the streets of Brooklyn had looked up, they would have seen a 13-year-old girl wearing a brace, hanging out the window of a 12th floor apartment. It wasn't smart. It was reckless.

But in those moments, as I did something I knew my mother would hate, I felt like I was in control. And I was never in control.

As I smoked, I'd think about the next day at school and the awful teasing I would endure. I'd think about the next weeks, and the next months, when I would be tortured some more. Doctors said I had to wear the brace for at least six months, 24 hours a day, or else.

If I didn't wear the brace, my entire body would collapse and fall into a mangled heap on the floor. At least that's how I translated what the doctors told me.

So I wore that brace religiously, just like I was supposed to, taunted every day at school. I endured the bullying, because I didn't want my body to crumble into a heap on the floor.

But then, one day, the doctors told me I could take the brace off when I was sleeping at night. Though if I got up to walk or use the bathroom or go anywhere in the house, I was supposed to put the brace back on.

One night, I woke up thirsty and I forgot to put on the brace before I walked to the kitchen to get something to drink. And I realized what I had conjured up in my mind was wrong. The doctors were wrong. I was walking through the house without the brace, and I hadn't collapsed.

I stood up straight and tall that night inside the kitchen, and I said to myself, "Forget this. Forget this dumb brace."

The next day, I went to school and I stuffed that brace into my locker, and I did the same thing every single morning after that. Sometimes I would sneak a different shirt to change into. It was always something very form fitting, something that didn't need to hide a big plastic brace.

> "She was supposed to wear that brace 24 hours a day. That was critical. But I did not know. I did not know that she was sneaking to school and taking off the brace. I feel very guilty that I did not supervise well enough, and she really suffered."
>
> —Sonja Lee, Jeanette's mother

I lost precious hours not wearing that brace. My spine didn't fuse properly after the surgery, and it didn't heal properly. Looking back now, I know how stupid that was. Scoliosis is a fierce opponent and if you don't address it correctly it will wreak havoc on your body.

I have paid greatly for not wearing that brace. There have been so many complications with my back since I was that middle school girl just wanting to fit in. So many surgeries and so much pain.

I've always wondered if I would've had the problems I had if I'd worn the brace like I was supposed to.

Most of my competitors and fans would say, "What problems?" Few knew, as I rose through the ranks of billiards, that I suffered from scoliosis, and even fewer knew how severe it was. I didn't want them to know. I didn't want to be pitied or be given an excuse for a bad game.

But after years of keeping my scoliosis a secret, I gave permission to my longtime friend and physician Don Wardell to "out" my scoliosis on pool's biggest stage.

It happened at my induction into the Women's Professional Billiard Association Hall of Fame in 2013. As Wardell gave my introduction speech, he talked about my pool accomplishments. At the time, I was 41 years old, had won more than 30 national and international titles, and I was ranked the No. 3 billiards player in the world.

"If you polled the people in any random meeting room, or any random person on any random street in any random city in the U.S., 60 percent to 70 percent would know the name Jeanette Lee, recognize it, and associate it with the sport of pocket billiards," Wardell said at my hall of fame induction. "In Korea, China, Taiwan, or the Philippines, the percentage is even higher."

Wardell went on to tell the room of people inside the Soaring Eagle Casino in Mt. Pleasant, Michigan, that I was an elite athlete who had persevered with a condition so severe, he wouldn't have believed it if he hadn't seen my X-rays with his own eyes.

"I knew Jeanette had been born with scoliosis before becoming her physician, and I assumed she must have a mild case," Wardell told the crowd. "After all, moderate or severe sciolous usually results in death or severe disabilities and, even with surgery, leaves the patient with limitations that usually prevent any type of sporting participation, much less the championship level of play like Jeanette pulled off while battling the disease."

And then Wardell told the room filled with pool stars from all over the world about my scoliosis and, for the first time ever, he revealed the cruel power it held over me all these years.

"She's overcome a condition so severe," Wardell said, "most medical professionals cannot believe that she has succeeded with such a condition."

When Wardell became my doctor, as I played the pool circuit, he obtained all my medical history, my X-rays, my tests, and records of my surgeries. He was completely shocked. He told me what I had done was the most amazing sports achievement he had ever heard of or encountered, and it changed forever the way he viewed me.

I have endured nine major surgeries for my scoliosis and pseudoarthrosis to prevent disability, paralysis, and even death. While I'm grateful that those operations that kept me alive and let me play pool, those surgeries also resulted in intense, chronic, debilitating pain.

The rods placed in my spine went from my scalp all the way to my tailbone. As I played pool, I always had two opponents fighting me, the opponent across the table and the opponent invading my back.

"I subscribed to *Sports Illustrated* for more than 40 years, and hardly a week would go by without some inspirational story about an athlete overcoming injury," Wardell said at my induction. "But in all those years, I have never read of anyone overcoming anything even as remotely severe as the series of surgeries that Jeanette has had."

To this day, I still struggle endlessly with back, sciatica, joint, and nerve pain. I always hope and pray for some relief. Just last year,

I had yet another surgery to implant a spinal cord stimulator into my body, a device that sends low levels of electricity directly into the spinal cord to relieve pain.

I'd had that device implanted before, and it was absolutely incredible, the wonders it worked on my body. For the first time in my life, I felt no pain. Literally, I felt zero pain.

It sounds silly, but when I came home from getting that device implanted for the first time, I was so ecstatic about my pain-free body that I started jumping on my bed. I was jumping off it, then back onto it, and then back off again. I was kicking my feet up in the air.

My three daughters stood in my bedroom, and they watched me in disbelief. To be honest, they were a little scared. They had never seen me do anything like this their entire lives. They were always acutely aware of my scoliosis.

"Mommy, stop!" they screeched at me. "You're going to get hurt! Mommy, stop!"

In my mind, there was no need to stop. That device inside my body was tricking my brain into not recognizing pain signals. Instead, it was focused on the pulsations and vibrations being given off by the stimulator.

"I'm free. I am free!" I yelled as I jumped on the bed. "Thank you, Lord."

That freedom didn't last long. Just days later, I noticed that there was white stuff oozing out of the surgical site where the spinal cord stimulator had been implanted, which soon became yellow stuff, which quickly became green stuff.

The incision from the device implanted in my body was not healing. I called the doctor, who told me this was an emergency situation. "Get in the car right now and meet me at the hospital," he said, "and pack an overnight bag."

At the hospital, they flushed the wound, and they cleaned it up. Surgeons put in quadruple stitches, promising me this would hold the device in. I went back home and rejoiced in that remarkable feeling of having no pain.

But five days later, I felt this weird feeling on my back. When I reached my hand to see what it was, my shirt was completely soaked. The wound was oozing again. I called the doctor.

"Jeanette, I don't think your body likes this thing," he said to me. The wetness on my shirt was spinal fluid dripping out.

Against my wishes, my desperate wishes to keep this device in and keep living a pain-free life, the doctor said it had to come out. He said that the spinal cord stimulator wasn't safe, because my body was fighting it.

I started crying, and I begged him, "Don't do this to me. This is the first time I've ever had no pain. You don't know what it's like. You literally gave me my life back. Please don't do this. Don't do this."

After a very long, emotional conversation, that doctor convinced me the device had to be removed. I remember looking at him and saying, "Okay, well, how long will I have to wait before you can put it back in?"

"I'm never putting it back in," he said.

I was devastated, but I forged ahead, enduring the extreme back pain that had been with me for 40 years. Still, I always hoped to one day have that feeling again, that feeling of jumping on my bed, completely numb, and carefree.

In 2024, I finally found a doctor who agreed to implant another spinal cord stimulator. I can't tell you how hopeful and desperate I was as I walked into the hospital for that surgery.

But, this time, when I came home, I wasn't jumping on the bed. This device was not reacting to my body like it had the first time. Some of the pain in my back was blocked, but not all of it. There was still a lot of pain, and that was an incredible disappointment.

My mind took me back to those days, all those years throughout my career, where the back pain couldn't be stopped.

The game of pool is difficult for a person without a disability. It takes dedication, sacrifice, and endless hours bending over a table. Scoliosis doesn't like bending over.

Tears would fill my eyes as I practiced night after night, as I fought to become better. I would wake up the next morning with stiffness so severe, I couldn't stand up straight for two hours.

I would literally walk around the apartment making breakfast, taking a shower, getting dressed, completely hunched over.

Because of my fused spine, I could not twist or bend at the table. It was impossible to reach those shots along the rail. I had a chronic, dull pain throughout my back and neck that only got worse as I bent to shoot a ball.

There were times I would stretch for a shot and get stuck in that position, unable to get up without someone physically lifting me off the table.

There were weeks and months at a time when I was not able to practice or play, even as my competitors were practicing and playing. I hated the idea that they were getting an edge on me. I would force my aching body to go to the pool hall and, within five minutes, I would have to quit because of the agonizing pain.

> "Even with scoliosis, when she was at the pool hall, she was maniacal in a way, or at least neurotic. She would practice and practice and practice and practice, 20, 22 hours a day until the other patrons, her friends at the billiards hall, had to carry her home weeping because her back hurt so bad."
>
> —Tom George, Lee's longtime manager

When I wasn't playing pool, scoliosis still followed me. I would go to the grocery store, lean over to grab a can of soup from the bottom shelf, and my back would lock up. I would have to call someone, anyone who would answer, to come to the grocery store and carry me out.

The customers would stare at me from the deli and the produce section. The cashiers would look on with pity. It was absolutely humiliating.

It didn't matter if I was at home, at the pool hall practicing, at a restaurant grabbing a bite to eat, or if I was battling in a high-profile tournament, there were always those moments when the pain became so intense, all I could do was cry.

But I always persevered. Every single time.

Before the finals of one tournament, I collapsed from back pain after winning the semifinals, and everyone counted me out.

> "She was in bad shape. She was in the bathroom, she was lying down on the floor, and her back was really going through spasms. But she got up, and then ran out and just played perfectly and won the [finals] match. So you know, she's a fighter."
>
> —Ewa Mataya Laurance,
> Hall of Fame pool player, in *Jeanette Lee Vs.*

Friends would always ask me why I sacrificed my health for pool, why I battered my body just to hit a ball into the pocket, why when the pain became debilitating, I didn't simply stop.

The answer was easy for me. I absolutely loved pool.

"Ask yourself, honestly, if you could have become a pro player in the face of such pain, in the face of such disability," Wardell said at my hall of fame induction. "The question of why Jeanette has persevered to develop this level of skill despite the pain and disability has always intrigued me. I truly believe it is because she loves the game, loves it so very much that all the pain and all the suffering is worth it."

Yes. Pool was always worth it for me.

Pool was what took me from a floundering soul to a woman who believed she could be a superstar. A woman who, despite all the surgeries and the intense pain, became the No. 1 pool player in the world.

But before I would become No. 1, before I would walk into Chelsea Billiards at the age of 18 and launch my pool obsession, I would first become a teenage demon.

I would become a rebel who fought every rule, and every person who loved and cared about me. And, as I did, I wondered why I couldn't be more like my sister, Doris, who, in my eyes and just about everybody else's eyes, was absolutely perfect.

I knew I could never be as good as Doris, so why even try?

CHAPTER 6

IN THE SHADOW OF AN OVERACHIEVING SISTER

I WAS NOT JEALOUS OF MY SISTER, at least that's what I tell myself now. I wasn't bitter toward her, at least I don't think I was. Doris was simply the yardstick with which I measured success as a young girl in Brooklyn.

And, in my mind, I always fell short of Doris. I was always walking in her shadow.

Doris was the first female idol I ever had. She was born in 1969 and I was born in 1971. Growing up, she was always two years ahead of me, always prettier than me, always smarter than me, always a better singer than me, and she had so much confidence.

I did not have confidence, not an ounce of it. I would follow Doris everywhere she went. She was like my barrier, a wall that protected me from the world. And she absolutely hated that.

> "When she was young—five, six, seven years old—we would go outside to play with our little gaggle of neighborhood

> kids, and I would treat her like a pest. 'Jeanette is following me. Stop following me.' Now I feel kind of bad, but I vaguely remember I would call her a 'dummy' or 'stupid,' and my mom would say, 'Stop saying that. Don't say that to your sister.'"
>
> —Doris Lee, Jeanette's sister

My mother didn't scare Doris, and she kept calling me names. But that didn't stop me from still wanting to be around her, still wanting to go wherever she went, and still wanting to do whatever she was doing.

I tried to be cool enough to be friends with Doris' friends. I tried to talk like she talked. She was perfect to me, so confident in her own skin.

I wished desperately that I could be more like Doris. I was never comfortable in my skin. I always felt like I wasn't enough—not smart enough, not pretty enough, not a good enough daughter. I definitely felt like I didn't fit in.

I just wanted to be like everyone else, anybody else, anybody but me. The neighbor girls in our apartment building were mostly Black, and I wanted their bodies. I wanted all those curves and cleavage.

I would stuff my barely-A-cup bra with socks, and I would wear thermal underwear underneath my Lee jeans to fill them out, to get rid of that gap between my thighs. I would look in the mirror and, still, I was never satisfied. I hated my body. Nothing about me was good enough. It was horrible.

No matter what I did, I never felt as pretty as those girls in my neighborhood. And I certainly never felt as pretty as Doris. She was beautiful and amazing, and she couldn't stand me. All I was to her was a bratty little sister, a wannabe Doris.

> "She always had a sort of envy or something of me which, you know, when you're little you just think, 'Ugh, my younger sister.'"
>
> —Doris Lee, Jeanette's sister

It sounds crazy but, even when Doris was yelling at me, I loved being around her. I just wanted to soak in everything about her, how beautifully she could sing, and how she played the piano so much better than I did. I was in awe of how easily things came for her.

Doris also had the most amazing fashion style in the whole world. I loved pretty things, cute clothes, and all her clothes were special. She never let me touch them or borrow them.

But when Doris wasn't around, I would sneak her clothes out of her room and wear them to school. When I got home, I would stuff them back in a corner at the bottom of her closet, hoping she wouldn't notice it missing.

Doris always figured out what I had done when she pulled out a wrinkled, worn pair of pants or blouse. She would erupt in a fit of fury and she would tell me how selfish and rude I was.

As her words came at me like darts piercing my soul, I knew she was right. I knew I shouldn't have taken her clothes. But when I wore her clothes, I kind of felt beautiful. More like Doris.

We did have some good times together, making snacks together after school, playing silly games, but Doris and I were just so different.

Mostly, we were the worst of enemies.

To me, it felt like Doris hated me, and that destroyed me; it crushed my spirit. She had no idea how much I looked up to her and thought the world of her, and she had no idea how much it hurt that she didn't reciprocate that.

We got into some major tussles, some pretty big rows, and some physical fights. We would pull each other's hair, bite, scratch, hit, punch, and pinch, the whole nine yards. I hated that she was so much stronger than me. It seemed like her punches always hit and mine always missed or just bounced off her. Even as I grew taller than her, I still felt weak against her. I never felt like I would ever win a fight and it made me both sad and angry.

I always, always felt like Doris was the golden child, and I thought she was my mom's favorite. As I was in the backyard playing rowdy games with the neighbors, Doris would stay in her room to read, sing, and study.

She would smile as she practiced the piano. I whined and complained. She would take my mom's side when there was a disagreement. I always took Doris' side.

My mom has always denied that Doris was her favorite. She says she had no idea that, growing up, I felt like I was competing against Doris.

> "In some ways, there was a rivalry between them. But, also, Jeanette was very smart, and she got her awards from the church, from the school. In some ways, they were a little different, but both of them were good at what they did, so I did not realize that rivalry [existed] very much."
>
> —Sonja Lee, Jeanette's mother

That rivalry resulted in me always feeling stupid compared to Doris. She was an academic genius.

In New York City in the 1980s, there was the option of going to a regular school in your district or taking specialized exams. If you were able to score high enough on those tests, you could be admitted to an elite academic school.

When Doris took those specialized exams, she was so brilliant that she was the first student in 17 years in our area to get into Hunter College High. It was a school on the Upper East Side of Manhattan with 1,200 students that represented, based on test scores, the top one-quarter of 1 percent of students in New York City.

Doris made it into that school, which has produced brilliant minds, including Ron H. Brown, the first Black man appointed to the Cabinet post of Secretary of Commerce in President Bill Clinton's administration. Another Hunter alum is world-renowned opera singer Martina Arroyo, who went on to be a Kennedy Center Honoree. So is Mildred Spiewak Dresselhaus, the first female officer in the National Academy of Science, who in November 2014, received the Presidential Medal of Freedom from President Barack Obama. Elena Kagan, the fourth woman to sit on the U.S. Supreme Court, also graduated from Hunter.

When I tried to get into Hunter College High, I failed miserably. As I took the exam, I sat shaking and sweating. I felt so freaking stupid. When the test was over, I remember crying because I knew I did poorly. I just didn't know the answers. I loved to read, but Doris read twice the books I did. I was twice as active as she was. I was good in school but I hated middle school and high school. I definitely wasn't Doris.

I was always too hard on myself. I know that now. I may not have gotten into Hunter, but I did get into The Bronx High School of Science, passing that exam with flying colors. I didn't lose a bit of sleep after that test. It was so easy for me.

People would tell me that getting into Bronx Science was a big accomplishment, that it was nothing to sneeze at, that it was a prestigious school, and that I should feel proud.

But, in my mind, Bronx Science wasn't good enough. It wasn't Hunter. It wasn't Doris' school.

> "Maybe she always had that feeling that I was doing that good-child thing, academically. But her personality was different. I tended to be kind of rational. I wanted things to

make sense. She's a little bit more emotional. After a while, our different personalities became even more clear."

—Doris Lee, Jeanette's sister

It wasn't just Doris' academic success that I looked up to. Doris did things I never could have dreamed of doing.

She would walk boldly down the sidewalk, never worrying what people thought about her. She didn't let the Korean slurs classmates spewed at us bother her. She just ignored them, though it twisted my insides up with anger.

I would often hear Doris singing along to music. It seemed like she could just listen to a song once or twice and immediately sing the lyrics. I always had a tough time separating the music from the lyrics. I would have to study the lyrics over and over to memorize them. That didn't come naturally to me. And it felt like everything came naturally to Doris. She was a girl wonder.

In elementary school, on the first day of classes, the teachers would say to me, "Oh, you're Doris' little sister." I knew what that meant. They were going to compare me to her, and they were going to be disappointed. I wasn't studious like my sister. She read all the time and had this incredible vocabulary.

I read, too, but it was usually Nancy Drew or *Encyclopedia Brown, Boy Detective* or books by Judy Blume or C.S. Lewis. Doris was reading deep stuff, genius stuff, and I felt like she was constantly judging me. She says I was wrong about that. Doris says she admired me.

I was smart, and I was in all the gifted classes, just like Doris, but she was the valedictorian of the entire school in sixth grade. She made it to the *New York Times* spelling bee and came in second.

I watched my mother beam with pride at everything Doris did. It never felt like she was beaming with pride at me.

I know it sounds like I was very jealous of Doris, but I wasn't. I admired her. I aspired to be like her. But as we got older, there were times she really got on my nerves.

Doris would come home from college when I was in high school and running away a lot, and she would see my mom and me arguing. Doris would shout, "Jeanette! Jeanette, how can you talk to mom like that? Stop now."

I would scream back at Doris, "Shut up! What do you know? You're not ever here. You don't know what it's like."

> "Some of the time when I came home, Jeanette was there, maybe not a lot of the time, but when she was, it would be intense, five-hour conversations, sometimes having a stupid fight over something. It was kind of intense."
>
> —Doris Lee, Jeanette's sister

As I was running away and trying to find my path, Doris was engrossed in creating a life of academic success. At the University of Pennsylvania, she majored in Asian studies, focusing on Japan, studying the Japanese language, its history, its art, and everything about its culture.

When Doris graduated from college, she came back to live in New York and worked briefly at a bank. Then she got a job as an assistant at Columbia University's library, which happened to have tuition benefits.

Doris enrolled in grad school and then earned a master's degree in the school of international and public affairs. In 1997, she moved to Hong Kong, looking for a job where she could use what she had learned in school and experience Asian life, our family's heritage, for the first time.

In Hong Kong, Doris reconnected with an old friend she had met when she studied in Japan during college. The two married and settled in Hong Kong. They had two children and Doris worked in banking, and then for a labor rights organization. In 2020, Doris received her Ph.D., and she is now a part-time lecturer at different universities.

As I made my living playing pool, and as Doris rose the ranks of academia, the distance in our relationship continued to grow. It hadn't really improved much since our childhood.

Doris doesn't remember it that way. She says the good times we had together far outweighed the bad.

> "We used to have fun sometimes, just rolling around doing silly things, playing like puppies. We used to have a lot of fun. I don't know why, but Jeanette has really negative memories."
>
> —Doris Lee, Jeanette's sister

Then, one day in my early twenties, while I was living on the West Coast, I received an international call from Hong Kong. It was Doris. She said she was just calling to say hello and catch up. I found that very strange; I didn't trust her. What was she trying to pull? Why was she calling me now, out of the blue, and acting suddenly interested in my life? We still saw each other over the years at holidays and family gatherings when she would come back to the U.S. to visit, but I would hardly call us close, and we certainly never called each other unless it was regarding Mom or Dad. I realize now that I was acting bitter and I should've just given her the benefit of the doubt and been more receptive. I knew Doris wasn't a manipulative person, so why pretend like she was untrustworthy? As annoying as I was to her—and she made that clear—I still always felt loved and protected by her anytime we were together. It was a pleasant conversation but I was skeptical. A week later, she sent me an email. She would ask how I was doing, how the weather was, and tell me about things that were going on with her. I replied to her with short answers and continued about my day. Then she sent another email the following week. Then another. She started calling me once a month and emailing me every week. I didn't know what was going on. It was pleasant but I really didn't share all that much about my life. But she never quit, so I started getting invested in the news of her life there. What was going at her job or at church or with her husband, Sidney, and her kids, Leni and Benji, who I adored.

When I received my Stage 4 ovarian cancer diagnosis, she was a saint, always calling to see how I was doing. She made doctor and therapy appointments for me and the girls. She listened to my concerns and offered ways to help me keep things in perspective. You see, I started having issues with my memory, which often caused me to struggle recalling simple words for things like a chair or a gas station or even being able to remember the name of a friend I'd known for 20 years. I was in so much pain, and on heavy drugs, both of which caused awful uncontrollable mood swings. I would snap at my poor girls, sometimes screaming in a bout of rage at my precious babies, who were already traumatized by my diagnosis. I was drowning in guilt. My longtime employee, Shylee, who'd become like a daughter to me, recently finished school and was excited to start her career as a phlebotomist.

The cancer and the chemo was horribly affecting my ability to run my business effectively. Thankfully, my APA consultant Jeff Hayes and my neighboring league operators, Mike and Sherie Strout, were incredibly supportive and kind enough to help me out for as long as they could. They had their own successful, therefore work-intensive, Bay Area APA business to run. The workload of running two successful APA businesses was taking a terrible toll on them. My battle with stage 4 ovarian cancer did not need any more stress and guilt. I didn't know where to look or if I'd find a buyer who would be a great league operator *and* love and treat my Tampa Bay APA members as well as they deserved. On top of all that, I'd never really gotten settled after the move to Tampa. There were boxes and bins piled up to the ceiling in the house and in the garage and even more in a storage unit.

I was trying to keep everything together, when COVID hit.

Then stage 4 ovarian cancer.

As close to Doris as I was, I was ashamed what a poor job I was doing on my own keeping everything together. It wasn't until I got my diagnosis that I really shared everything that had been on my mind. In the end, when it looked like every door was shutting around me, Doris, my *Unni*, stepped through and took on *all* of it.

Today, I am very close with my sister, and I am thankful to Doris for developing our relationship.

As I face terminal cancer, things like that matter so much more to me now, those family ties, family roots, true friends and, of course, my children.

My six children, their spouses, my grandchildren, my godchildren, they all mean the world to me. They are my everything. And I pray every day that they will never feel the insecurities I felt.

I pray they will never want to run away from me the way I ran away from my mother, breaking her heart as I raised hell.

CHAPTER 7

"GOTTA RAISE SOME HELL BEFORE THEY TAKE YOU DOWN"

I TURNED INTO A HEADCASE somewhere around the age of 13. I blame it on the body brace I had to wear for scoliosis at the time, which resulted in dark thoughts invading my mind. They were very negative thoughts, feelings of no self-worth, feelings of hopelessness. My life seemed absolutely miserable.

I had been raised a Christian. When we were little, my mom would send me and my sister Doris to Bible camps in the summer. I would sing the hymns, read the verses, and pray. I loved the idea of God, this epic, spiritual being who, I was told, only wanted the best for me.

By the time I was 13, I had a hard time believing God wanted the best for me. I had a hard time believing there could actually be a God who loved me.

Yet, I still prayed to him in earnest. I pleaded with him: *God, why are you doing this to me?*

My mom would always say to me, "Don't worry, Jeanette, God has great plans for you. Everything happens for a reason. This is God's plan. Just trust in Him."

I would look at my mother and tell her to shut up. "You don't even know what you're talking about," I would say. "You can't understand what this is like. You can't feel what my body is feeling right now, and you can't know what my life is going to be like."

> "Jeanette was unbelievably unhappy. She used to have such a sweet smile, and that was totally lost. It was gone."
>
> —Sonja Lee, Jeanette's mother

My mother was right. I was unbelievably unhappy. Wearing that big brace, I felt like an ugly ogre. I didn't understand why I had to be a girl with scoliosis. I didn't understand the torture, so I turned against myself.

Scoliosis destroyed me, not just physically, but mentally. It destroyed any positive self-image I had, which wasn't much to begin with. I used to be a pretty happy kid, in general, always wanting to make people happy. That was gone.

I became a dangerous mixture of insecure and rebellious, and it made me easy prey for an older family friend who would kiss me when my parents weren't around.

As he pulled me toward his body and put his tongue inside my mouth, I wondered what was wrong with me. Feelings of shame set in.

I can admit now that I suffered trauma as a child, but I never thought of it as me being abused. I was too young. Probably around six to nine years old. I know it's hard to believe, but I never made an issue of it because it didn't continue and because I didn't think it affected my life in any way. It was just something that happened. I'm bad about downplaying trauma in my life. I don't want to shame my family, and I don't want to ever be called a victim.

But that family friend who lived in our apartment would lure me into a dark room, and he would kiss me. I was in elementary school, and he was in college. It's not like he was some 40-year-old, gross middle-aged man, but he *was* a man, and I *was* a girl, and he should not have been kissing me. Thankfully, he moved away, so it stopped.

Years later, as I played pool, rising to the No. 1 woman in the sport, it became obvious that people thought I was pretty, but when I looked in the mirror, I still saw the scrawny, little girl with thick glasses and awkward posture. Of course, as any young woman, I wanted to look my best, but I certainly didn't have confidence in the way I looked. Not after the way I grew up. I always seemed to only focus on the negative things I heard people say. I grew up never fitting in and was made fun of for my looks.

But in the beginning, when the veterans of the WPBA and the media were spreading rumors of how cocky I was, I didn't think anyone thought of me as special, or better than anyone else. I didn't really get why so many guys were looking at me or noticing anything special.

I was just me. And, in my mind, I wasn't anything special at all.

I was just Jeanette, a girl who'd been sexually abused, a girl who had been taunted for being Asian and bullied for being too skinny, and a girl who grew up always wondering why her biological father had left her.

And in middle school I became the girl who started hanging out with the wrong crowd.

Around the time of my scoliosis diagnosis, my mom had saved up enough money to buy her very own house. We moved out of that towering apartment building in Brooklyn to a two-story home in Bayside, Queens. For my mother, she had truly achieved the American dream.

I feel terrible now that my bad behavior, my running away, my delinquency, ruined what should have been a very joyful, celebratory time for my mother. Instead of reveling in the pride of the beautiful home she had made for her family, my mother was spending every minute worrying about me, what I was going to do next.

When I was in seventh grade at I.S. 391 (Intermediate School 391), in Crown Heights, Brooklyn, I would get into fights. The kids were always making fun of me, so I fought back. I was so small compared to my classmates that they could have blown on me and I would have fallen over. I came home, day after day, beaten up.

One day, when my mom visited the school after yet another fight I had gotten into, she saw used condoms and bloody tampons in the stairwell. That was the last time I walked into I.S. 391.

My mother promptly moved me out of that school and enrolled me in Elisabeth Irwin High School, a private academy in Greenwich Village in Manhattan, which included grades seven through 12. My mom thought that school would be good for me. It was not good for me at all.

Moving me to Elisabeth Irwin, my mother always said, was the worst mistake she ever made.

I might not have gotten beaten up at my new school but, at Elisabeth Irwin, I started pushing my boundaries with boys. I started cursing like a sailor. And I started trying drugs. The students at the private school had money, and that meant access to more things, some of them bad things.

One of those students was a girl who I thought of as a best friend. I really thought she was the coolest girl I'd ever seen. I think it was because she was so confident. I wanted to be just like her. She was the most amazing thing in my life because, for the first time in my life, I finally had a best friend. I absolutely idolized her.

She was a punk rocker with a mohawk who thought rules were made to be broken. She listened to the Sex Pistols, who belted lyrics like, "Don't know what I want/but I know how to get it."

We would hang out at Central Park from the afternoon into the wee hours of the night. I cut off my long black hair and wore black clothing. I had a camo green jacket that I cut off at the sleeves and wore every day. I painted my entire room metallic black, got a black lamp with a red bulb, and my life turned very dark.

My friend and I would take needles and punch holes in our ears. I was always a wannabe who easily gave in to peer pressure. One day, my friend decided that we should become blood sisters.

She took a razor blade and cut her wrist a couple of times, and we watched as the blood started squirting out. When she gave me the blade to cut my wrist, nothing happened. I started squeezing my arm like crazy and, still, no blood.

So, I cut again, and I cut again, and I cut again. It took 28 slits before we actually saw blood. By that time, we were laughing hysterically. We pressed our wrists together, mixing the blood, and became sisters forever.

When the wounds on my arm started to scab up, I wore long-sleeve shirts to hide what I had done. But one day my mom saw the ugly red scars. They horrified her, and she was furious. She lectured me and she told me how disappointed she was in me.

Luckily those scars were the only outward, telltale signs of all the poor choices I was actually making.

It was around that time that my mother really started losing me. I was very resentful of her. I only focused on what my mother was not, instead of what she was. I didn't feel like I had a relationship with my mom where I could talk to her. I often felt invisible, as if she never understood me, and I didn't know how to express to her what I was feeling.

My mom loved me, she cared for me, she worried about me, and I always knew that. She was a woman who only wanted the best for me, but I didn't see that at the time. I saw the glass half empty, and so I got my attention elsewhere.

I smoked weed for the first time at Elisabeth Irwin. I learned how to blow smoke rings with cigarettes, three packs a day of Marlboros. I thought I was unbelievably cool, and I felt even cooler when my friends praised me. No one seemed to understand what I was going through, except for the crowd I hung out with at school.

By the time I got to The Bronx High School of Science at the age of 14, I was a true delinquent. I cut classes and smoked weed all the time. I was lost. I didn't have a reason to wake up in the morning. I was just living, drudging through life, and disappointing my parents.

When I was younger, I had big plans to please my parents. On the first day of first grade, my teacher gave us our first homework assignment. We were to write down what we wanted to be when we grew up. I couldn't choose between growing up to be an artist, an actress, or a teacher. But I knew those careers would make my parents happy.

In high school, I was very far away, light years away, from that little girl who wanted to please her parents.

I tried acid for the first time when I went with some friends to a Yes concert. I hated the way the drug made me feel. I started going crazy, seeing weird things, kind of hallucinating, and it scared me to death. I never tried acid again.

By the time I was in high school, my parents and I were very distant, very far away from one another. We didn't have the kind of relationship where we would talk. I couldn't tell them how insecure and sad I felt.

They were always working, so I was always sneaking away, even after my mom gave up her nursing career to be home with me.

> "I was very worried, and I quit my job to be with Jeanette, but she would not let me. I stayed at home and tried to pay attention to her. But I realized it was too late. She was too much doing her own thing, and so I was running behind her, rather than leading her."
>
> —Sonja Lee, Jeanette's mother

After my mother quit her job, I felt suffocated. On Saturday mornings at 8:00 AM she was downstairs in the basement of our house where my room was.

She would pull open the drapes covering the windows and yell at me to get up. She would tell me I was wasting my life. It drove me crazy. I was used to raising myself, to my mother not being around, to having no rules.

My mother would tell me to clean up after myself, that there should be no trace of me left behind. Put everything away, wipe down the table. I never did things as well as my mom thought I should, so she would show me how to do them, and then make me practice wiping down the table right in front of her.

My mom did her best to discourage my bad behavior by trying to instill faith in me any way she could, any way she thought I could relate to.

My great-grandfather had been a minister, and my mother would always talk about how grateful she was for him, her grandfather. She was so proud of his faith and devotion to God, and she had such fond memories of getting up each day to have morning worship with him. She wanted me to feel that way about God.

I had a pet albino ferret named Jumper that I absolutely adored. I had gotten him when I got my first studio apartment as a teen, on 23rd and Lexington. He was so cute, but he smelled horrendous. He invaded my tiny space with putrid, noxious odors. It didn't bother me because he was so cool and I just loved that little thing. Jumper went everywhere with me.

My mom would tell me the way I felt about Jumper was how God felt about me. "That feeling of love you feel for your ferret? That is God," she would say.

She would make Xerox copies of Bible verses and use Scotch tape to plaster them to my door, so I would see them when I came home from a late night out. She would constantly ask if I believed in God, if I was acting the way God would want me to.

> "I would tell Jeanette, 'Respect God.' But she was angry with me and would tell me, 'I'm not happy. And if I'm not happy, there is no God.'"
>
> —Sonja Lee, Jeanette's mother

I never stopped believing in God, no matter how unhappy I was. It was more a feeling of anger about the hand I'd been dealt. I didn't care if God was watching all the bad things I was doing, watching me disrespect my mother. I was just pissed off all the time, at least whenever I was home. I really don't know why.

My mom and I have a good relationship now, but we did not when I was a teenager. We had a very bad relationship. There was the time I was beaten and mugged and my mother slammed the front door in my face.

In her mind, I'm sure, she thought I had gotten what I deserved.

The mugging happened when I was barely 17 years old. To get to New York City from our house, we had to take a bus and three subways. One night, after being out very late, I was coming home at 3:00 AM, got off the bus, and took a shortcut, walking behind houses on a dark, dead-end street.

I was on my way home from a photo shoot. A friend had told me I should try modeling, so I did. I was walking briskly toward my house, carrying a big satchel full of my nicest clothes. I didn't have many nice clothes but, for the shoot, I had brought my favorite, prettiest clothes.

As I crossed the street, I noticed a car idling behind me, and then the car drove past me. One of the guys got out of the car to smoke a cigarette. Three other guys got out and were just standing there. I knew immediately this wasn't good.

I started walking really fast down the street, my head down, and the next thing I knew those guys were jumping me. As they grabbed my bag, I pulled back with all my might, screaming for them to let go. One of them said, "Shut up, bitch."

As they snatched my bag and started running toward their car, I ran after them and jumped headfirst into the driver's seat. I was getting those keys out of the ignition, because I was going to get my bag. I was not going to let them have my prettiest clothes.

Instead, those guys started hitting me. They beat the living crap out of me, threw me on the street, took my bag, and drove away. But as they were driving away, I took a mental note of their license plate number. They may have gotten my pretty clothes, but I was going to bust them.

I got up in excruciating pain and hobbled toward my house. When I got there, everything was locked up. I started pounding on the door for what seemed like hours. Finally, my mom came downstairs, opened the door, looked at me, and she slammed that door right back in my face.

I pleaded with her, trying to tell her I had gotten mugged, but she had already gone back to bed. At that point, my mother had definitely had it with me. I don't blame her. I was a teenage delinquent, staying out all hours of the night, hanging out and doing whatever I wanted. She had no control over me and it must have been exhausting.

Eventually, my uncle, who was visiting, let me inside, and we called the police. My mother didn't even come downstairs to be with me as the cops helped me file a police report. Because I had gotten the license plate number of the car, all four young men were arrested—though the police never recovered my belongings.

But the attack had left me with a dislocated hip, a sprained neck, and a broken heart. My mother had shown me, in my mind, that she was done with me.

> "I blame myself for those years that I lost that affected her life somehow, and I cannot make them up."
>
> —Sonja Lee, Jeanette's mother

Soon after the attack was when I moved into my own studio apartment, and I eventually got a job as a receptionist at a Korean computer company, filing papers, answering phones, editing reports, and organizing things at the office.

When I turned 18, I also worked nights as a waitress at a rhythm and blues lounge called Tramps, which happened to be owned by the same guy who was opening Chelsea Billiards across the street.

It was at Tramps that I met Barbara Wong, a hostess at the club, who became the first real, true, close friend I ever had. When I would hang out with my friends in high school, I never really knew what they thought about me. I never really knew what they said about me when I wasn't around.

I didn't wonder about any of that with Barbara. She was genuine and I trusted everything about her. Barbara had gone to Hunter High School, where Doris went, and they had been friends there but they hadn't stayed close. They were very different. Their friendship was more surface level, but Barbara and I hit it off right away on a much deeper level.

Having Barbara in my life, I felt a new sense of safety and support. She believed in me in a way no one else ever had. She always saw the good in me. We became inseparable.

After our shifts, we would go to 24-hour diners, and we would sit there for hours talking into the wee hours of the morning about our dreams. Barbara wanted to be an attorney and was feverishly studying in law school.

I remember thinking how incredible that was. Any spare second she had in between hostessing and taking tickets at Tramps, Barbara would be reading her law books.

I soon became obsessed with playing pool across the street at Chelsea, and Barbara and I didn't get to see each other as much. Still, she would always stop by the pool hall to visit me. She never made me feel guilty for our lack of time together. She was constantly telling me how brave and strong I was. With all my insecurities, I didn't believe her at first. But eventually I realized that courage and strength is forging ahead in the face of doubts and insecurities, not the lack of them. For some reason, she always believed in me. I don't know why, because I certainly didn't think I was special. I was just really determined. But Barbara was the first real friend I truly had, and she would just marvel at how dedicated I was. I felt the same way about her. Now she's a successful immigration attorney and partner at a law firm in Fresno, California.

When I took a break from Chelsea Billiards to follow my then-boyfriend up to college at University of Buffalo, Barbara would write me letters about how proud she was of me. I never felt deserving of her support. It was wonderful, but I always felt guilty that I didn't visit her more often. We always stayed in touch and we always promised one another that when we got older, we would live close enough so our kids could grow up together.

Barbara and I always reminded me of the two characters in the movie *Beaches*, which starred Bette Midler as C.C. and Barbara Hershey as Hillary. I was C.C., the more wild and rambunctious of the two, who was an aspiring actress. Barbara was Hillary, a straight-laced, conventional type, who wanted to be an attorney. They were two completely different people who forged an unlikely friendship that endured through the years.

That was Barbara and I. No matter where our lives took us, we remained best friends. She was the maid of honor at my wedding. When I was diagnosed with cancer, she came to stay with me. We reminisced about our days at Tramps, how as Barbara diligently studied law, I did some crazy things.

There was the night I first tried cocaine. My boyfriend, Greg, who had been my high school sweetheart, had started using the drug so, of course, I had to try it, too.

It was the opposite of weed. It made me focused, smart, strong, tough, cool, and fun. Everything in life was wonderful when I was high on coke, but that was also a problem. I felt invincible and, growing up in New York, I knew that wasn't right. No one was invincible.

This was one of those times in my life when I think God intervened and helped me. I became scared of the feeling coke gave me, and I also had a gut feeling that this was very wrong. I knew that every time I did it, I wanted more. I never went and bought my own cocaine. I only did it when Greg and I would get together with his friends.

But after just a few times, I knew I had an addictive personality and cocaine seemed like a feeling that should not be legal. It was dangerous. I envisioned myself completely destroying my life and selling my soul.

I'm not sure what gave me the willpower to say no to using cocaine again, other than God and pool. I had just started playing seriously, and I knew I was heading down a bad path that would disrupt my dreams of getting better at the sport.

I also gave up smoking pot because of pool. One night before going to the billiards club, I smoked weed with my friends. As I practiced at the table, I hated how ineffective I was. I decided then I needed a clear mind if I wanted to really succeed at this newfound love.

To be honest, I feel like pool saved me from myself. Pool saved my life.

It was the only addiction that ever stuck with me, an addiction to green felt tables and cue balls. I went from being a lost teenager who wanted nothing more than to raise hell, to becoming absolutely obsessed.

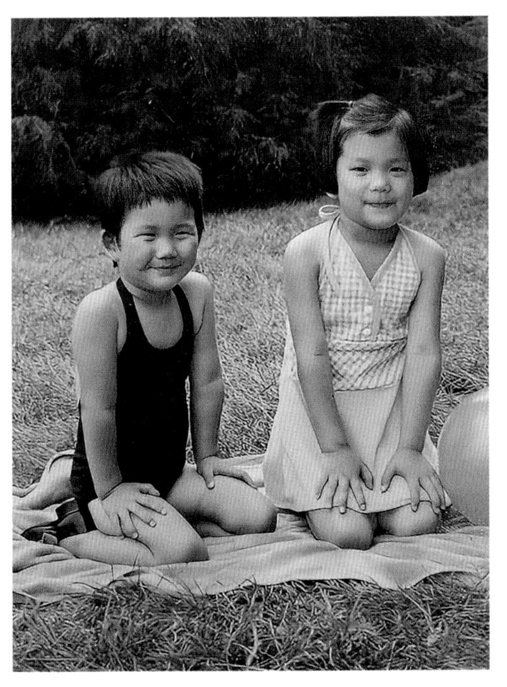

Here I am at two years old with my big sister, Doris, who was four.

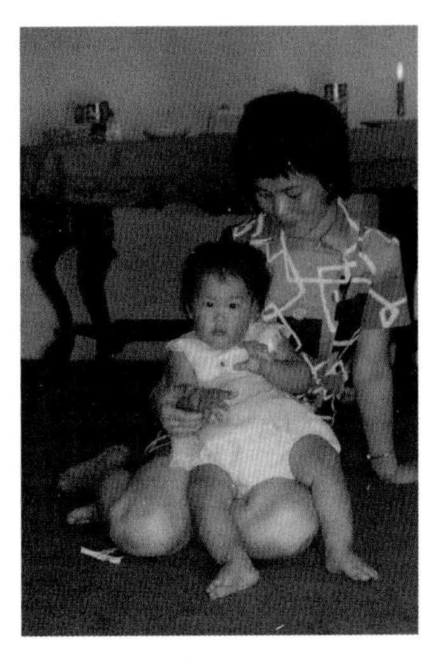

My mom and I.

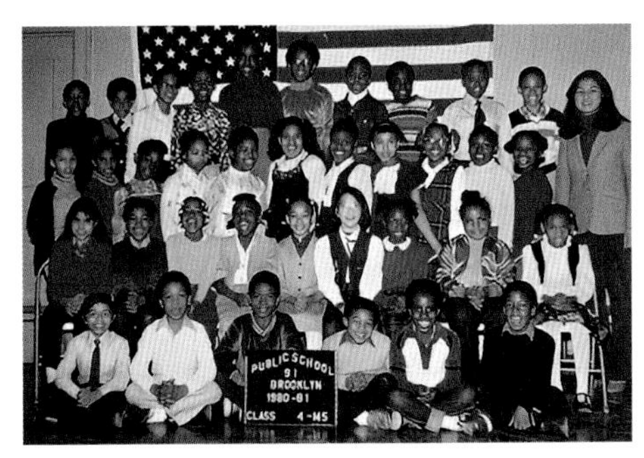

My fourth-grade class photo with Mrs. Chin, my favorite teacher.

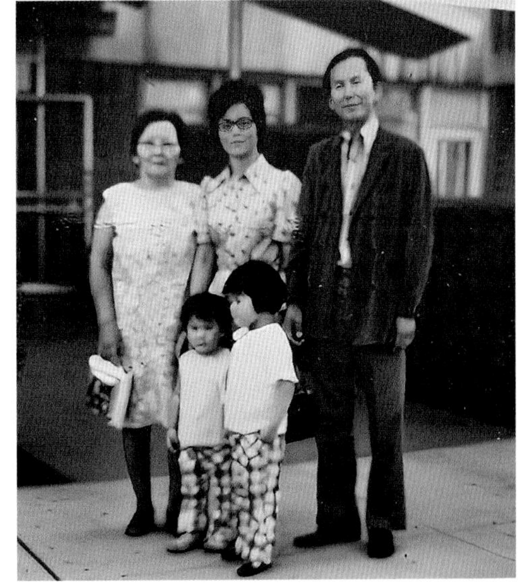

My paternal grandmother, my mother and father, Doris, and I.

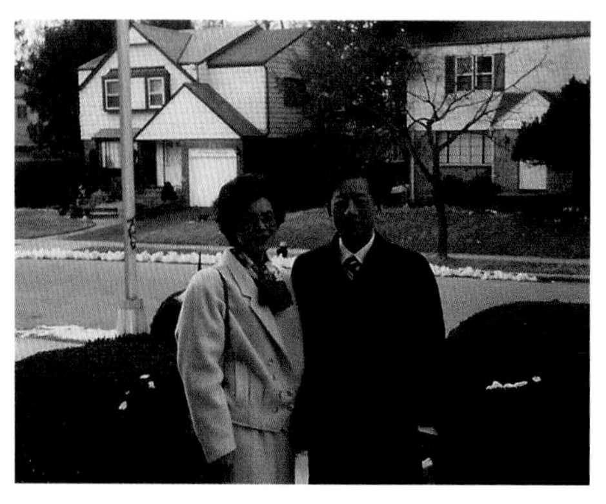

My mom and dad after they moved us out of our Brooklyn co-op, to our first house in Bayside Queens, living the American dream.

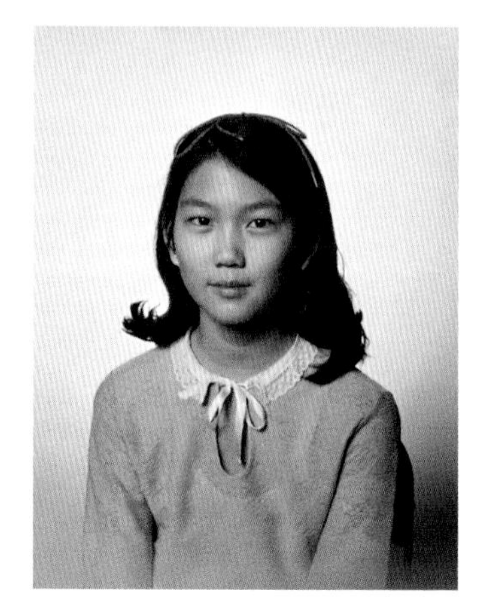

Here I am at 10 years old.

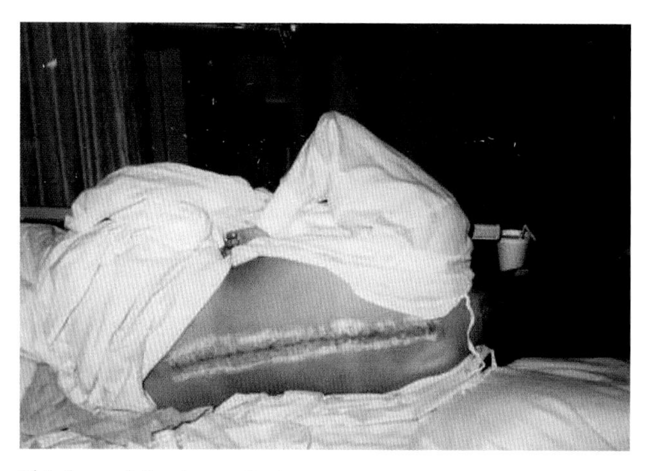

This is me following scoliosis surgery.

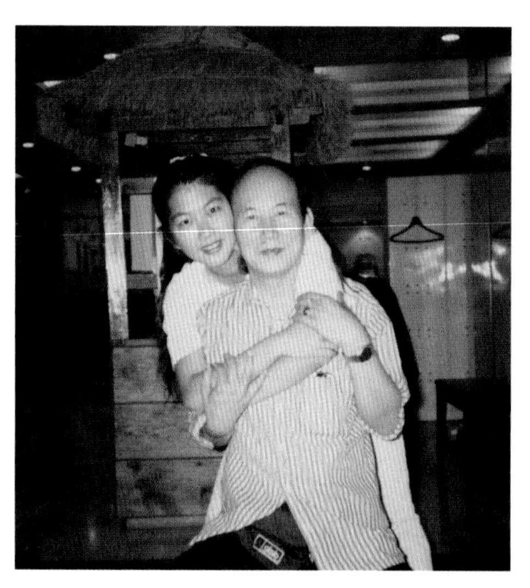

Reunited with my biological father, John Tak, when I was 19 years old.

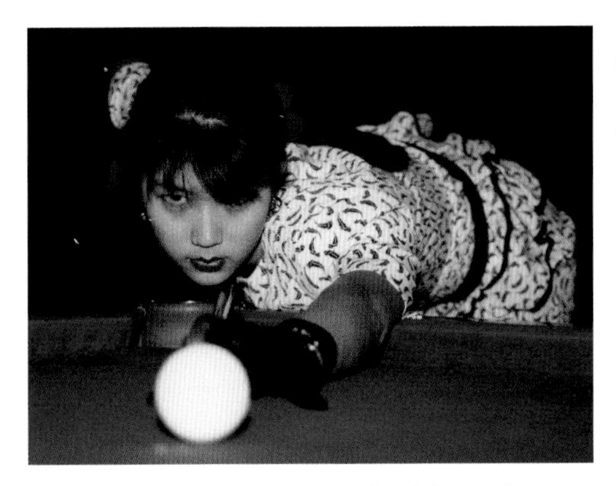

This was at Amsterdam Billiards Club. By this time I was already known as one of the best women players in NY. I didn't have the Black Widow nickname yet. This was one of very few dresses that I had. I must have been around 20.

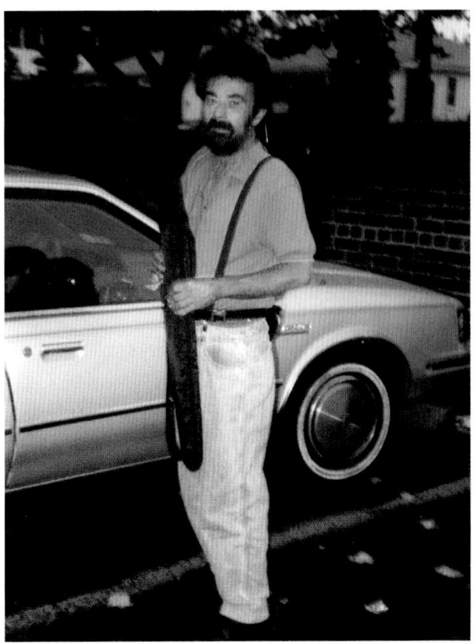

Gene Nagy when I first met him.

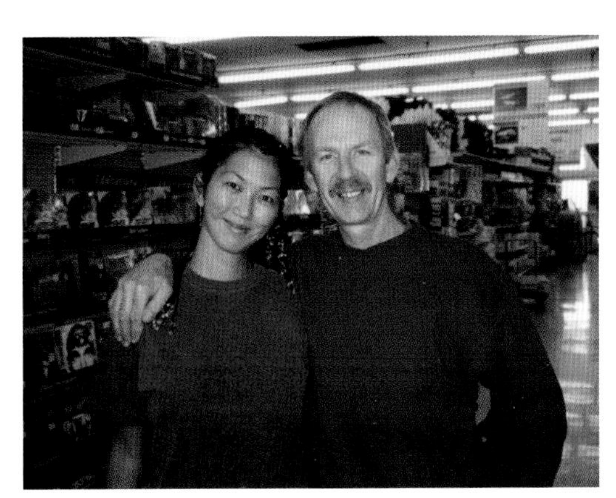

Early years with my coach Bob Carman.

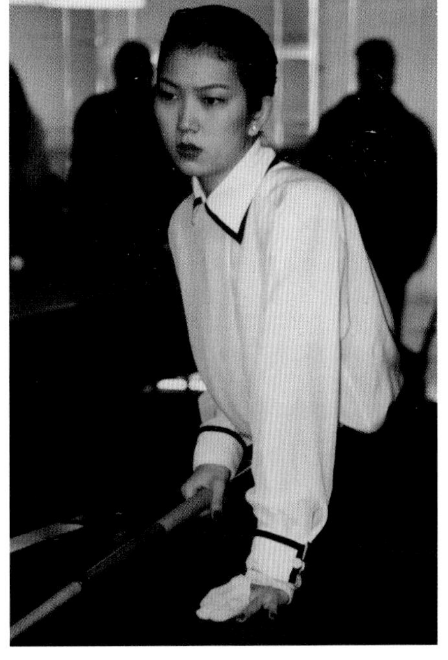

Me at my first WPBA Classic event in 1993. *(Courtesy of Billiards Digest)*

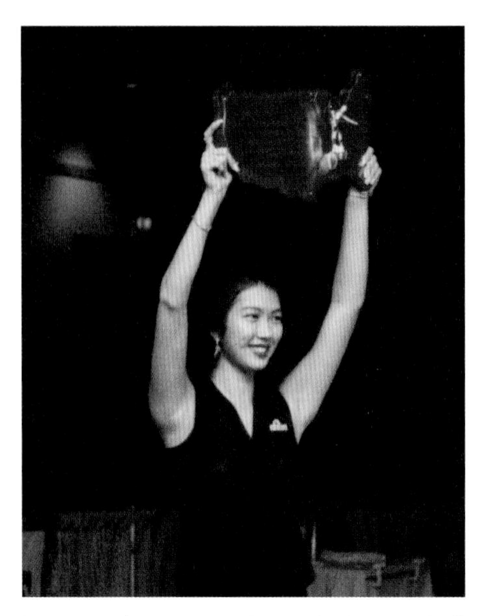

Winning the 1994 WPBA U.S. Open 9-Ball Championship. *(Courtesy of Billiards Digest)*

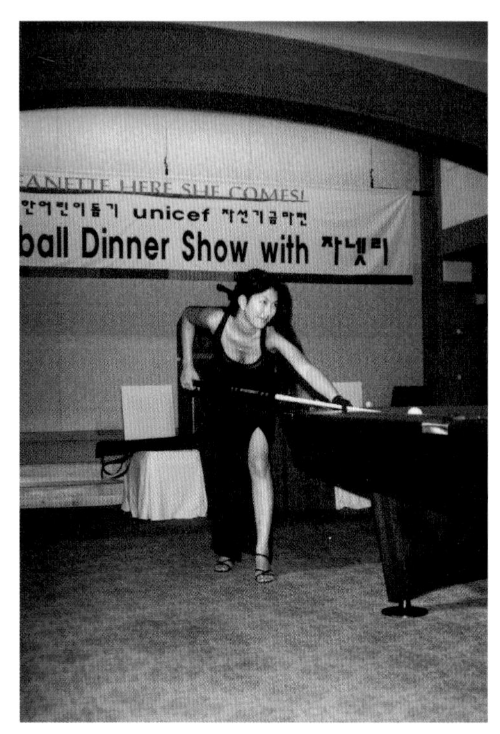

I did a big tour with my manager, Sunny Kim, in Korea. It was a great experience and my second time in Korea after my first time when I was 19. It was so different because this time, I came as a star. They rolled out the red carpet and chauffeured me everywhere. I loved being so well received but I was ashamed that I wasn't more fluent in Korean.

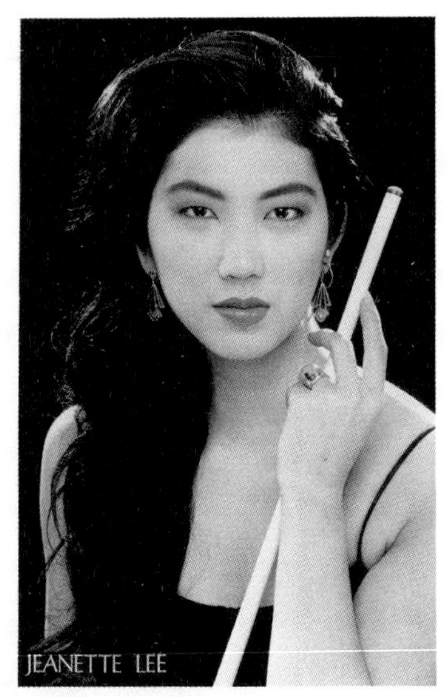

Howard Beach Billiard Club. *(Courtesy of Billiards Digest)*

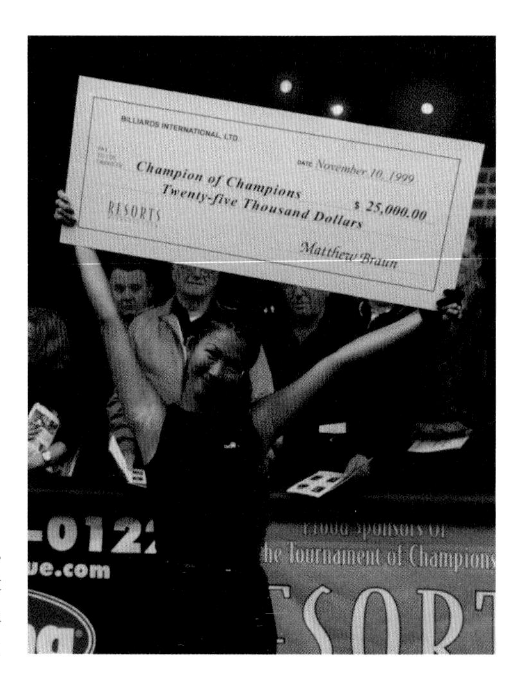

I won the Champion of Champions in 1999, which was a $25,000, winner-take-all tournament comprised only of women who had won a WPBA Classic Tour event.

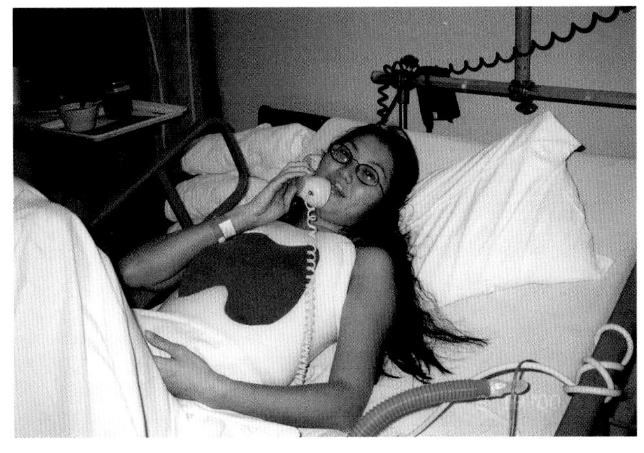

This photo is right after my back surgery. I had neck, shoulder, and back surgeries, each three weeks apart. Just after the surgery for my back, I got a call informing me that, as the top American, I would be representing the United States for the first time ever for billiards as an Olympic sport in the 2001 World Games in Akita, Japan. I was panicked because I'd finally get my chance to compete for a medal, on a stage that recognized a variety of sports, and I would not be prepared—at least, not as prepared as I would've hoped.

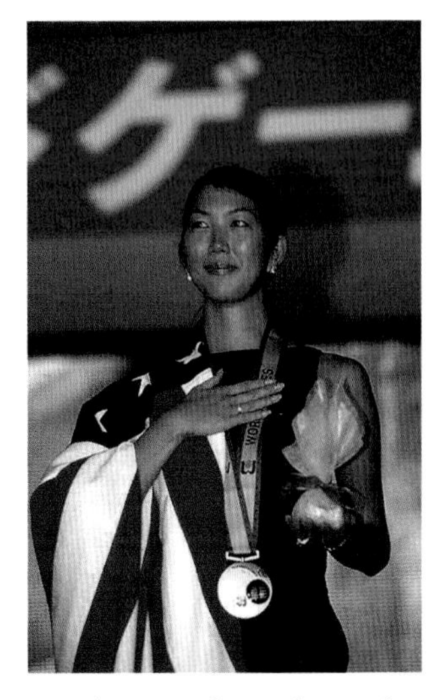

Standing on the podium after winning the gold at the World Games. Truly, the greatest experience I ever had.

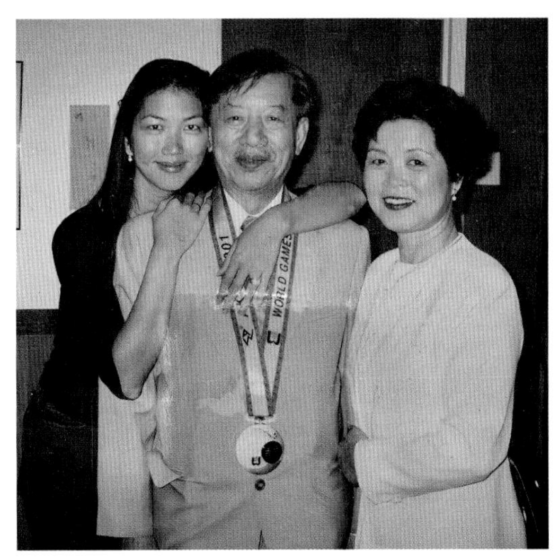

I finally brought home the gold for my dad.

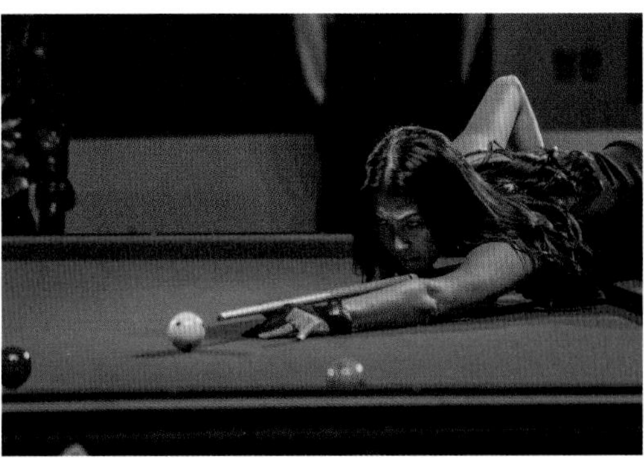

Playing during a match in Goyang, South Korea. *(Seung-il Ryu/NurPhoto via AP)*

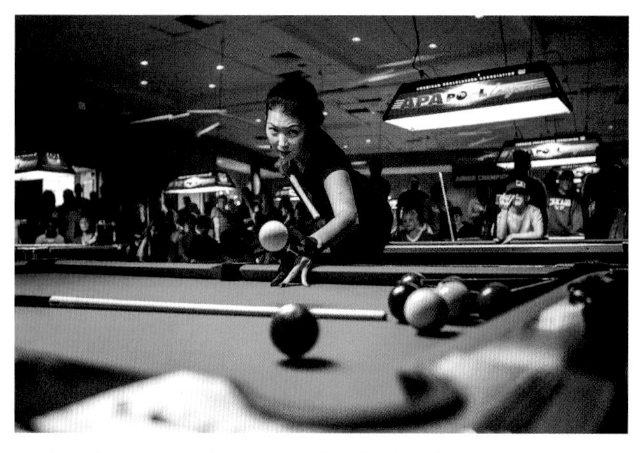

Performing a jump shot at an APA National event.

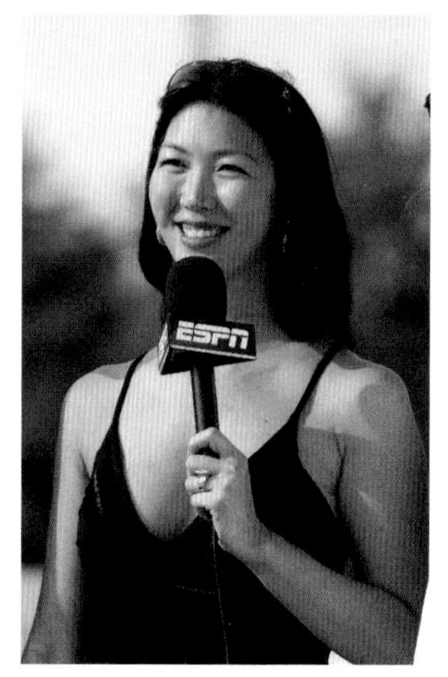

Here I am hosting for ESPN. *(Bill Greenblatt/UPI/Newscom)*

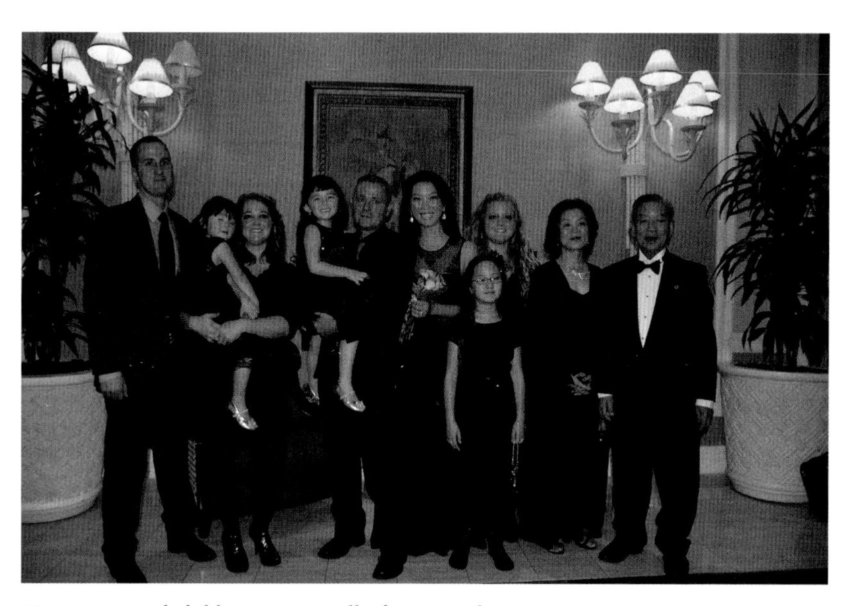

My parents and children at my Hall of Fame induction.

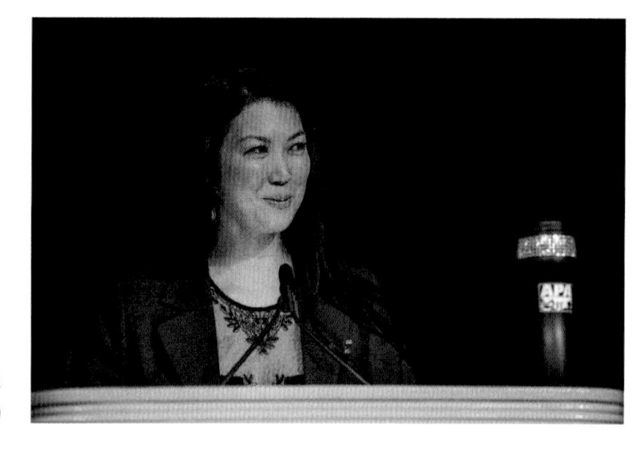

Speaking at my Hall of Fame induction banquet. *(Courtesy of Billiards Digest)*

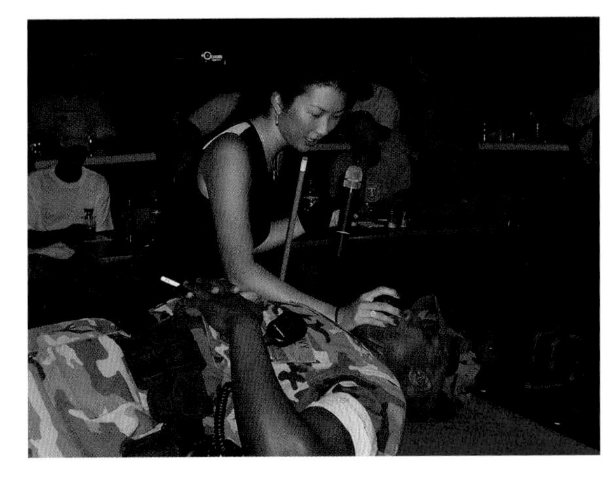

Entertaining the troops overseas. I liked laying a man over the pool table, resting the 8-ball on a piece of chalk held between their teeth, and resting a cue ball on four pieces of chalk on the wood rail. Then I'd shoot the cue ball in the air at the 8-ball and it would fly down to the far corner pocket. The crowd goes wild.

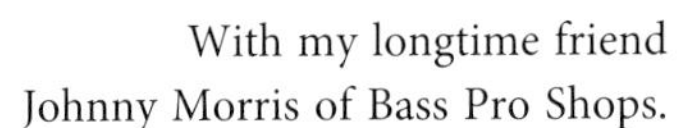

With my longtime friend Johnny Morris of Bass Pro Shops.

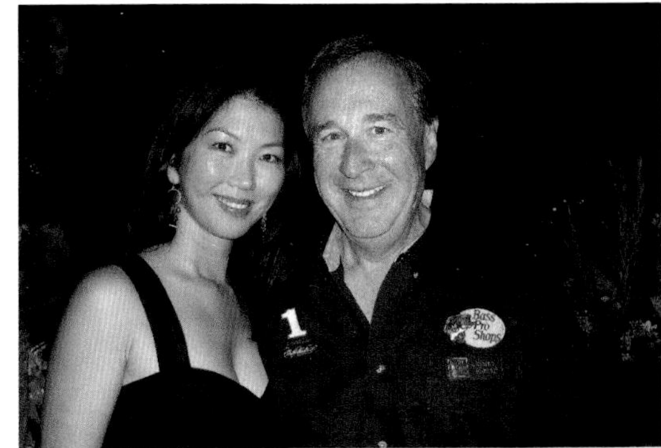

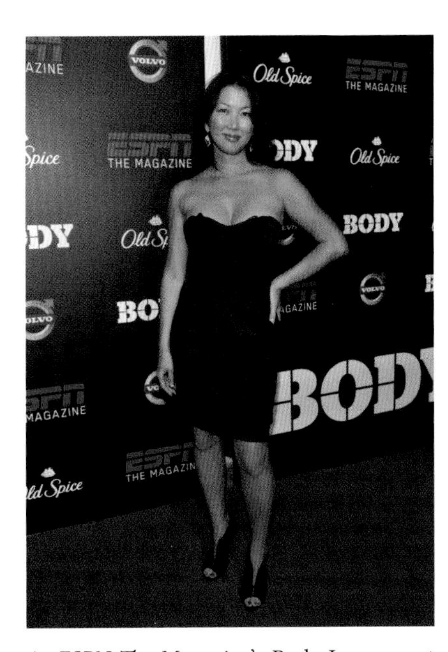

At *ESPN The Magazine*'s Body Issue event in New York in 2010. I had literally just given birth to my daughter Savannah, but I could still fit into that little black dress! *(Henry S. Dziekan III/Stringer/Getty Images)*

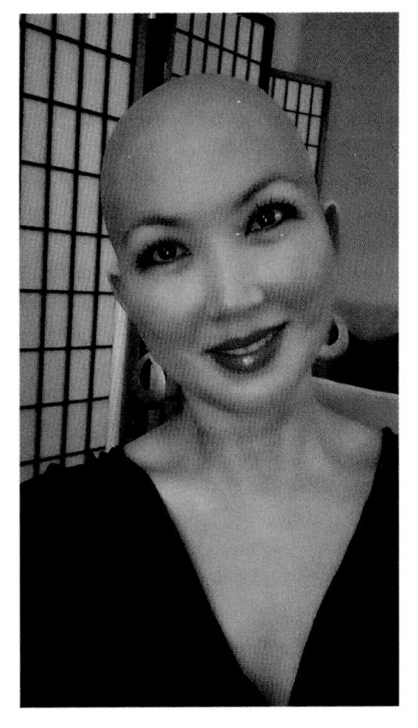

The first photo I took of myself after all my hair fell out. That same day, I made the announcement of my cancer to the world on my Facebook page.

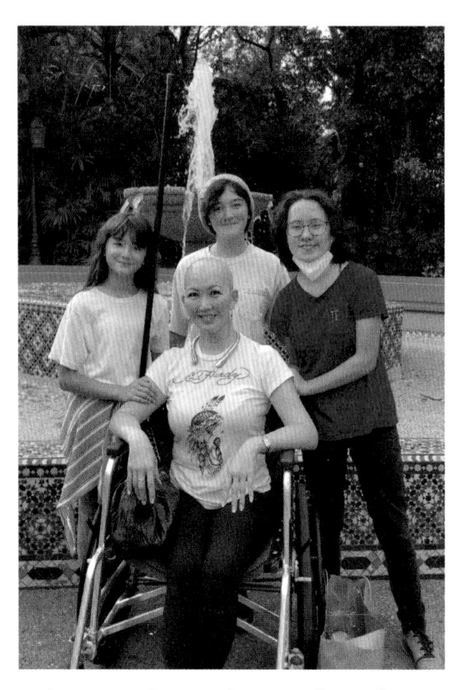

A day out with my girls at Busch Gardens.

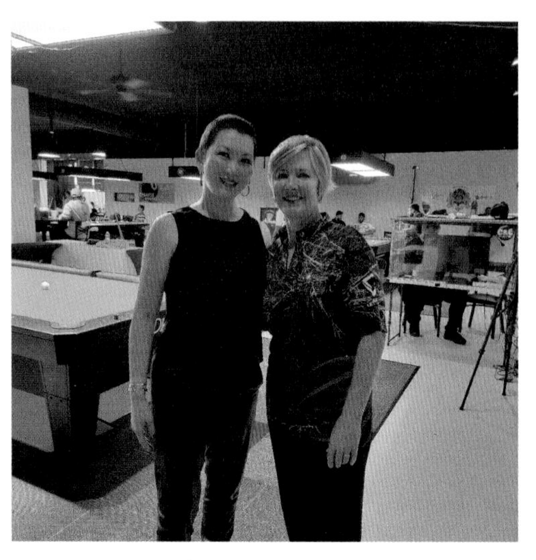

My nemesis, my friend, Allison Fisher.

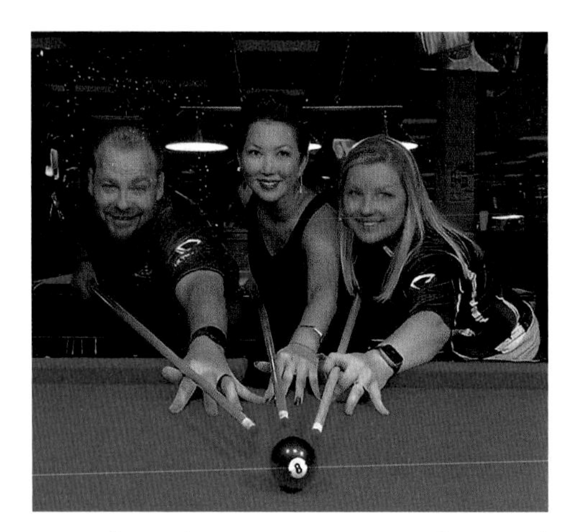

Me with my business partners, Anthony and Stephanie Spano of Tampa Bay APA.

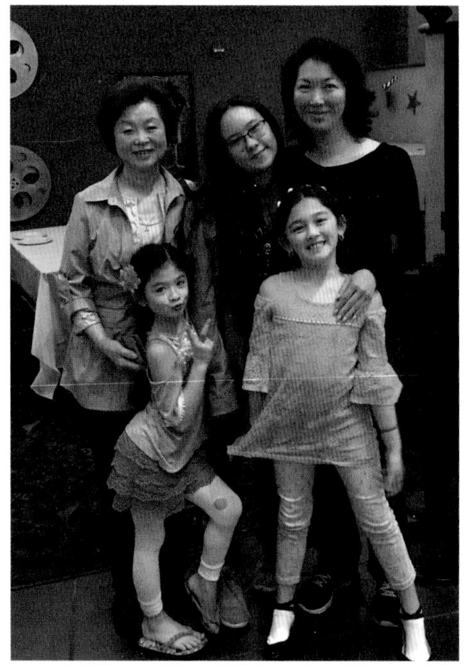

(Clockwise from top left) My mom, Cheyenne, me, Chloe, and Savannah.

CHAPTER 8

THE OBSESSION: "IT WAS LIKE AN OUT-OF-BODY EXPERIENCE"

I WASN'T EVEN SURE why I existed before I started playing pool. I wasn't sure why I was here on this Earth, a place that was rarely wonderful and, more often than not, pretty terrible. I wasn't sure what my purpose was in life.

When I found billiards, something that I finally truly loved, everything changed. Suddenly, I had a reason to care about myself, to be the best version of myself. Pool was an escape from all the things that made me unhappy.

Some people use drugs or alcohol for that escape. Pool was like a powerful drug to me, an absolute addiction. I had tried drugs before, but not even cocaine gave me the kind of high that pool gave me. It was an out-of-body experience to control a table or to come with that impossible shot when everything was on the line.

Part of the freedom I felt playing pool was that it was the first time that all of my insecurities seemed to disappear. I was able to focus my mind in a way that gave me a break from this big, bad world that I lived in. It was the first time I didn't care about what anybody thought about what I looked like or who I was. Before pool, I was miserable because I felt like a misfit and didn't have a purpose.

I was so obsessed with improving my game that I found myself rarely looking up. I didn't even care whether anyone was watching me. There wasn't time to think about whether I had a good or bad life—I was only thinking about how I could improve my game faster.

My pool addiction began when I was 18 years old, and I walked into Chelsea Billiards, and I saw pool magic. I was enchanted and captivated and it seemed like time stood still.

There was, of course, George Mikula, the older guy in the far back corner who was a wizard at the table. But there were guys gambling and hustling for money with names like Skeeter, Spanish Eddie, and Blood, which I thought was exciting. And there were very few women players, which I took as a challenge.

I went home that first night after 15 hours of watching pool at Chelsea, went to bed, and I dreamed about what I had just witnessed. I had never seen the game of pool played like that.

> "She was confident, strong, and determined. I thought she was so cool. I admired her tenacity and courage. Although she was beautiful, she was not just another pretty face. She had so much drive and grit. She was a great waitress and so sharp and fast. She always worked hard and money seemed to come so easy for her. I remember one of the nights at Tramps, John F. Kennedy Jr. came into the bar and she played a game of pool with him. Jeanette was an awesome friend, and she would always stand up for me. She was so smart and she knew what she wanted. There were so many boys around that wanted her attention and time, but her focus was always on pool. She had a poster in her apartment

> on the door that said, 'Master the cue ball and master your life' or something like that. She was on fire for pool and wanted to practice and excel. All the other stuff she was doing for money was just peripheral."
>
> —Barbara Wong, Lee's close friend

I came back the next night to Chelsea—and the night after that and the night after that. Soon, I realized my day job was taking too much time, but I still needed money. I wasn't about to ask my mom for it. The owner of Chelsea opened a bar across the street called Tramps. I started working there as a waitress; the money was better in less time. That's where I met my first real friend, Barbara. She was just a couple years older than me, Asian, and beautiful. We became close friends really quickly but I was on a mission to be the greatest pool player and she was studying law. She would often come to Chelsea to visit me and that made me feel really special. I was there every single day, every single minute I could be there. I eventually took all kinds of jobs, trying to figure out a way to work less and play more.

I always felt like every minute I wasn't practicing pool that all my competitors were gaining on me. I thought that as long as I was playing billiards more than they were, as long as I was playing while they were eating out at restaurants, or going to parties, or going to movies, I was gaining on them.

That's the mantra of most elite athletes, trying to find a way to get an edge on their competitors. Swimmer Michael Phelps, the most successful and most decorated Olympian of all time with 28 medals, once told the story of how he got his edge.

Michael and his coach, Bob Bowman, figured out that if Michael swam each Sunday for a year, that would add more than 50 training days that his competitors would be missing.

> "So they were always playing catch-up. I was just getting that much further and further and further and further away."
>
> —Michael Phelps

The work ethic of Serena Williams, the former No. 1 women's tennis player in the world, always resonated with me, too. Widely considered one of the greatest tennis players of all time, Williams was never shy about revealing just how hard she trained. She would practice endlessly, overnight into the wee hours of the morning, for hours straight.

Williams even had a court built at her home to replicate the court at the U.S. Open, with the official tournament surface installed. She always wanted to get an edge on her competitors. In interviews, she would say things like, "Don't let anyone work harder than you," and, "If I don't get it right, I don't stop until I do."

> "Luck has nothing to do with it. I have spent many, many hours, countless hours, on the court working for my one moment in time, not knowing when it would come."
>
> —Serena Williams

When I needed to take a break because of my back pain, I would sit and watch the other guys intently. I would analyze their shot selections and cue ball positioning, comparing what I would do with what they actually did. I was not a spectator watching to see who won; I was mentally playing the table. I paid attention to every little thing the players did. This helped my knowledge of the game grow quickly.

If I was driving, I would put my hands at ten and two on the steering wheel, both of them in the bridge formation, as I drove. If I was on the subway, I would practice the perfect swing along the edge of a row of empty seats. I would stroke my arm, trying to make sure my wrist was directly under my elbows. I didn't want to have any flaws at the table.

When I went to bed at night, I would fall asleep playing pool, picturing myself at the table. At first, I would just break the balls, then I would just try to make the balls. I was very, very, very bad. I played miserably. You would think that in my imagination I could play better, but I didn't.

Yet, each night as I fell asleep playing pool, little by little, I got better at controlling my mental imagery. Eventually, I was clearing the table in one inning. I was playing better in my mind than I was at the table in real life.

I'm not sure anyone can grasp or possibly understand my absolute obsession with pool. Even I have a hard time trying to explain it.

I can only compare it to the character Fast Eddie Felson, played by Paul Newman, in the 1961 movie *The Hustler*, who was on a mission to challenge and beat pool icon Minnesota Fats, played by Jackie Gleason.

That movie was about Felson's quest to be the greatest pool player of all time. He had a psychotic passion, almost a sickness, and that's who I identified with. I identified with Felson's need to be the greatest.

As far as I'm concerned, my hard work and dedication to the game were virtually unmatched. In all of my years competing in pool, I can only think of two other players who put in the effort I did.

One was a guy named George SanSouci, who was nicknamed "Ginky." He and I started playing seriously at Chelsea around the same time, and I was always just a little bit better than him. Ginky refused to play defense, so I would usually get him in the end.

I had an on-again/off-again boyfriend named Greg who was going to college up at SUNY Buffalo. This was my high school sweetheart and at the time I believed we'd be together forever. I didn't want to work odd jobs forever, and I missed him so much, so I followed him up there and enrolled in college, figuring I could still play pool there. Big mistake! I did play pool there, but it was at the student union with bad billiard tables and not much competition. Eventually, after a few more breakups with Greg, I decided to move back to New York.

When I got back to Chelsea Billiards a year and a half later, Ginky was one of the best players in New York City, rivaling the likes of Tony Robles, Frankie Hernandez, and Sammy Guzman.

Ginky was impressive; he played around the clock. He not only learned to play defense, I watched him practice the same bank shot for hours on end. He'd practice breaking the balls and then immediately rack them again, break them again, rack them again, over and over for hours. He showed so much discipline. He was the hardest-working pool player I had ever seen, until I met Karen Corr, who became one of the greatest women to ever play the game. Karen is the only player who ever swept the women's tour, winning every event in a single year. It was an absolutely incredible and astonishing feat.

Sadly though, even with her unheard-of accomplishment in women's billiards, Karen never picked up a single sponsor. She was painfully shy. She wore big glasses and oversized blouses to hide how big her breasts were. The WPBA had hired makeup artists and wardrobe stylists to help players who made it to the final rounds of a tournament look more stylish, but no matter how many times she reached that level, she was always too uncomfortable to make such changes. She hated doing interviews or having to do any trick-shot exhibitions to entertain the crowds. She just wanted to improve and let her game do the talking, so that's what she did. She was the first person on the practice tables at tournaments and she was the last to leave.

But with all of her successes, it was still too expensive to go on tour without sponsors. It was hard to make a good living. The prize money wasn't high enough and, eventually, Karen stopped competing. I always thought that was one of the greatest shames. We lost a great player, a great role model, a good person, and the hardest worker I'd ever met, all because she wasn't deemed marketable enough.

I have seen so many people with natural talent who never became great because they took it for granted and didn't work hard enough.

Of course, I had a certain amount of natural talent, but I didn't bank on that. I relied on my relentless work ethic and focus, my almost unworldly ability to notice all the little things, all the minute things.

I don't have a photographic memory. It just seemed like I did because I paid such close attention to what was happening, both on the table and off of it. I felt like everything mattered. Every little thing mattered.

When I would watch someone play, I would take in their breathing, their walking, their elbows, their grip hand, their bridge hand, their stance, their tempo, their force at the break, their subtleties. As a guy would take a shot, my eyes would follow his eyes.

Years later, after becoming the No. 1 pool player in the world, I would watch matches with my friend and fellow pool player Helena Thornfeldt, and it would blow her mind.

At one tournament, I watched one of our competitors at the table who had a straight-in shot. As she was down stroking her cue to shoot, I jumped out of my seat and told Helena, "Oh my gosh, she's going to miss."

Helena looked at me, laughing, and said, "What are you talking about? It's a straight shot."

I had noticed that the player had shifted her back foot, which changed her alignment and also indicated that she wasn't focused. Her mind was on something else. I knew that nuance wasn't good, and I was right. That player missed the straight shot and Helena looked at me in amazement. "How did you know that, Jeanette?"

My ex-husband, George Breedlove, was always amazed, too, by my attention to detail. He always told me I would dominate at poker. Of course, poker wasn't the game I wanted to dominate at.

Every night, after I played pool at Chelsea Billiards, as I walked home alone to an empty studio apartment, I would worry that I would forget how to play while I was sleeping. I obsessed over perfecting that bridge, the one the guys used, that allowed me to rest the cue right between my thumb and my finger.

At first, I used electrical tape to secure my hand in the bridge position while I slept. But sometimes I would wake up with my hair stuck to my hand. I quickly switched to masking tape.

I wanted that hand position to be automatic. I wanted it to be where I woke up and, boom, my hand was in that bridge, so that when I got to the pool hall, it was already familiar to me. Not just familiar, but second nature.

I may not have been able to play like a pro yet at 18 years old, but I was going to make sure I looked like a pro. I knew I would get better so much faster if my mechanics were like a pro and not like some amateur.

In my mind, it was always, "How fast can I learn this?" because I wanted to be great. I wanted to be the greatest. I was on a mission to become the No. 1 women's pool player in the world.

In the beginning, the early months, I was annoyed by my own incompetence. I was annoyed by how long it took me to actually start making balls fall into the pockets. It was a grind, but I was obsessed with it.

Any free moment I had, I was at the club. Sometimes I would practice for 20 or 30 hours straight. I would clench my teeth as I bent over the table, trying to overcome the indescribable back pain from my scoliosis. I knew I should stop. Instead, I kept playing.

There were nights my friends at the billiards hall would have to pick me up off the table where I was stuck in a position I couldn't get out of. They would carry me home as I sobbed in misery. I would wake up the next morning, forget the hell I had been through, and go back to the pool hall. There was just something about the game that sucked me in. I was a prisoner to pool, a prisoner who didn't want to escape.

By the time I was playing every day at Chelsea, I was a Bronx Science High School dropout who had earned my GED and was enrolled in college. Growing up, I always knew I wanted to work with children, so I majored in elementary education and early childhood development.

But as I played against the men at the pool halls, I wasn't sure I wanted to go to college anymore, especially after I started entering small tournaments and winning—winning against some really big names.

> "She came to me and said, 'I play with some top players and, occasionally, I win. I'm ready to compete with them. I can always get college, but this is the right time to join pool. Otherwise, I may lose the chance.'"
>
> —Sonja Lee, Jeanette's mother

I started playing in a lot of weekly tournaments where the entry fees were $20 to $25. If you won—and if you were lucky—you might get $500. I didn't care about the money, other than the fact that I needed that money to enter more tournaments.

There were different levels at those tournaments, A, B, and C. When I was only good enough to play the C level, I played in the B level. When my game rose to the B division, I played in the A division. I would usually get my butt kicked, but that was good for me. It seasoned me for taking any hit that came my way.

I was never intimidated by any player I took on throughout my career because, as an amateur, I was putting myself up against the beasts.

Tony was known as one of the best all-around players in New York City. His moniker as the "Silent Assassin" suited his quiet but deadly game. I'd been copying people my entire childhood, and now he was who I wanted to mold myself after. I studied everything about him. I watched him in every tournament I could. He rarely showed much emotion, but his elegant style and businesslike disposition made it hard to look away. I thought, "Why can't I be like that? Why do I always have to be so emotional? I wanna be cool and brilliant like him." I sure tried. I tried my best to emulate him, to stop being so hot-headed and stay calm and emotionless. It was hard and I tried for two months. Every time I missed my shot, I kept a poker face and sat down. Inside, I was steaming; I was constantly so angry at myself for missing such easy shots. I played awful. I thought, "Okay, Jeanette. Just be patient. Tony didn't become the 'Silent Assassin' overnight. Just keep it together and never let them see you sweat." One weekend, I signed up for a big tournament and off I went. I played awful. To be honest, having a poker face and trying to walk smoothly and decisively around the table didn't have the effect on my game I'd hoped. I felt like I had a straitjacket on and couldn't breathe. I felt like a cold, empty shell. As I walked from shot to shot, I felt dead inside. Where was my firepower, my heart, my competitive spirit? I realized that I'd squashed it by trying to be something I wasn't.

A lot of the women on the local circuit wouldn't play in the higher-level tournaments, because they didn't think they were good enough. I always wanted to be the underdog. I wanted to get in there and be competitive.

I didn't like losing, but I didn't mind losing. I knew when I was losing to a better player, it was like getting a free pool lesson.

Whenever I would win prize money, whether it was $8, $80, or $800, that money went to pay the entry fees for more tournaments. That's all I cared about. I had no need for anything else, no earthly or material things.

I had to be No. 1 in the world. I was driven by the idea of becoming No. 1, because I knew that was it. That was the pinnacle. But in my quest to become No. 1, as I struggled to get the money I needed to enter more tournaments, I did something pretty terrible.

To this day, it is the worst thing I have ever done in my life.

CHAPTER 9

LURED INTO A WEB OF DECEIT AND CRIME

AS A 19-YEAR-OLD FLEDGLING POOL PLAYER, I was always struggling for money, and Jake the Snake knew that. He was one of the most intimidating characters at Chelsea Billiards. He was a monstrous guy who always wore a long trench coat, a signature hat, and sunglasses, even when he was inside the pool hall.

It seemed like Jake the Snake was always at Chelsea, every single day, just sitting and watching. He never said much, but he was a standard fixture inside the club. The only time I really saw Jake talk, or even move from his seat, was when some sort of action took place around the pool table, some outrageous hustle, or a big gambling showdown.

Jake the Snake was daunting, kind of frightening, and unbeknownst to me as he watched me play pool, he had big plans for me. Illegal plans.

I have never publicly talked about any of this. I have never talked about the worst thing I ever did in my life. I've hidden this story for more than 30 years.

I was terrified that the illegal scheme I pulled off with Jake the Snake would end my pool career.

> "It's a secret Jeanette guarded for years because it was embarrassing. It still is a little embarrassing, but now, enough time has passed that she's allowed to have some peccadilloes in her youth."
>
> —Tom George, Lee's longtime manager

I was targeted by Jake the Snake because I was young, pretty, and Asian. I never knew Jake's real name, but he knew mine. And he knew Jeanette Lee was the wild child of her family, a bit of an outcast, and he knew I was short on cash.

My mom certainly wasn't giving me money to pursue this eccentric dream I had of playing pool for a career. She hated everything about it. She desperately wanted my love of billiards to dissipate so I could finish college and settle into a secure, ladylike career.

When I met Jake, I was adamant I would one day be the best player in the world. But I was nothing more than a menial laborer working odd jobs, and table time wasn't free. Jake the Snake knew that.

As I practiced day after day, paying for all that pool time, my mother would ask me how I was able to practice so much with so little money. I had learned pretty quickly that while I didn't have the cash to gamble, nor was I good enough yet, there were plenty of nice guys willing to play me for table time.

We'd negotiate a game, sometimes with a handicap, and the loser of the match would have to pay the table fees. That loser usually wasn't me.

As my game improved, I did eventually start gambling, betting small money—$10 or $20 a set. That's all I could afford. But little by little, those winnings added up as I started cashing in match after match after match. I could win $200 on an average day, and up to $1,000 on a really good day.

From the beginning, I was always able to outsmart almost every cat in the pool hall. Sometimes, it would take just a few minutes at the table to win a $20 bet.

As I look back on those games now, I don't know if I truly was winning, but I'm pretty sure to this day that my victories were legitimate.

I was a woman, after all. And my gender was always enough to make the men bet poorly on what they thought I could do at the table. They thought for sure, no problem, no sweat, that they could beat a woman. They would underestimate me over and over and over again, no matter how many times they watched me run out and win.

I may have been beating the men at the pool hall, but those small money bets never created a life where I felt financially comfortable. I was never way ahead. I never had a stockpile of money stashed away in savings. I always had just barely enough to cover my table time and barely enough to just gamble a little bit more.

If only I had more money, I would think to myself, I could bet higher. And I could win more.

One night, after 15 hours of paying for pool time, I turned to a friend and started talking about how I wanted to start playing more regional tournaments. I lamented how I rarely had the extra money for travel expenses. "Man, I need to make some money," I said.

Jake the Snake overheard me, and he jumped at the chance. He wanted to help me.

"You want to make some quick, easy money?" Jake said to me. "You meet me tomorrow, at 34th and Broadway, 11:00 AM and you'll make some real good money."

That seemed innocent enough. Maybe Jake had some players for me to gamble with. I soon found out that wasn't what Jake had in mind at all.

When I showed up at 11:00 AM the next day, Jake promptly escorted me out the door. He took me on a walk around Times Square. "Listen to me, if you do exactly what I say," he said to me, "you can make $1,000 today."

What? A thousand dollars was like a million dollars to me. I was all in on this seemingly fabulous gig.

Jake walked me to a building I didn't recognize and took me up the stairs to a room full of people I didn't recognize. He told one of them to photograph me. That seemed odd. I immediately felt like something shady was going on.

But I still posed in front of the camera, just as I was told to do, as Jake stood with his arms crossed, blowing puffs of smoke. There was no way I could say no to Jake. *No one said no to Jake the Snake.*

After my photo was taken, we all sat there hanging out, making small talk, until, suddenly, things moved very quickly. Somebody walked in with a credit card and an ID, someone else's ID. But they had cut out that person's photo and replaced it with a picture of me.

I had a fake ID, and I didn't like this at all.

I tried desperately to think of a way to get up the nerve to back out. But Jake was looking at me in a way that said, "You better not change your mind now."

Jake was a bad dude. He was a dominating figure, a large Black man who wore an overcoat and sunglasses, who always had a cigar hanging out of his mouth.

I was scared. What had I gotten myself into? I didn't feel good about what was about to happen, even though I had no idea what was about to happen. Jake was intentional in what he told me, telling me just enough, but not enough for me to understand that I was about to do something illegal.

Jake sent me with another girl, a Black girl, to Macy's on 34th Street. I was told to walk up to the counter and buy a stash of electronics using a check from the checkbook in my wallet that also held credit cards and a driver's license, that fake ID that had just been crafted.

My chest was pounding as I ordered those electronics, and the anxiety and panic only grew as we walked back, carrying the stolen merchandise up the stairs to where Jake was in that building. We finally made it to safety and sat the goods down in front of Jake. He smiled.

I know now that Jake had targeted me for his illegal scheme because I was Korean. I was of great value to him because everybody in his circle was Black. And, as wrong as it was then and still is today, Black people are scrutinized more than a Korean woman, especially when buying a horde of electronics.

Jake knew the salespeople would be a lot less likely to question an Asian woman than a Black person coming in to make a large, expensive purchase.

After my first illegal deed on that very first day, Jake paid me $1,000 in cash, just as he had promised. He told me he wanted me to go back to another department store the next week, and do the same thing again.

I tried to rationalize what was happening. I didn't have to do this forever, just a few more times, and I'd have plenty of money for pool. I wouldn't have to work as many hours at my other jobs.

Deep down, though, I knew it wasn't right, and I didn't want to do it again, but I was too scared to tell Jake I had changed my mind. Now he had something on me, something evil I had done. If I backed out, would he kill me? I already knew too much.

I wanted to escape Jake, but I thought there was no way I could escape him. Chelsea Billiards was my house, my home pool hall, and Jake knew that. He knew he had me just where he wanted me, because he knew where to find me.

But Jake didn't know there was a savior in that pool hall looking out for me, a savior named Sammy Kong.

Sammy was one of the regulars at Chelsea Billiards, a guy I really looked up to. He would come in and practice and, occasionally, he would practice with me. While I was working to become one of the best women players around, there were a lot of big money matches played downstairs in the basement at Chelsea.

Every week, there was a regular, straight pool match between Sammy and Tony Robles for $500 a game. Back then, I didn't usually watch other matches. I always wanted to be playing, not watching. But when Sammy and Tony would play, I would sometimes go downstairs to watch them, to soak in their billiards magic.

They played with class, patience, style, focus, and respect for the game, and respect for each other. Sammy and Tony were the guys I wanted to model myself after. Until I met and watched Efren Reyes, Tony was my favorite player in the world. He was such a good player, but I loved how calm he seemed at the table, whereas I was so emotional. I'd get so mad at myself every day for making such careless mistakes and not improving as fast as I wanted. I didn't have anything to compare against, so I was very hard on myself.

One night after practicing for hours, just a few days after I'd gone to Macy's with a fake ID, I was ready to leave Chelsea when Sammy came up from downstairs. We practiced for a couple more hours, but my back started hurting, and it was 5:00 AM, so I told him I had to go home.

As I was leaving, Sammy asked if I was hungry. I was starving. He asked if I wanted to go out to eat with him. The only place I could think of that would be open was a 24-hour diner on 23rd Street. Sammy asked me if I'd ever had French food. I had not.

I'm pretty sure, as I look back now, that God was looking out for me. It was rare that I would leave Chelsea with a man to go do anything. But that night, when Sammy asked to go to dinner, I said yes. I don't know why I said yes. I only knew Sammy as a regular at Chelsea, but I trusted him, and I was starving.

We hopped into a cab and went to a French restaurant that, for some reason, was open. As we sat there at the dinner table, Jake was on my mind. In just a few more days, after all, I was supposed to meet Jake again. Do I keep going along with his illegal scam? What will happen to me if I tell Jake no? It was really bothering me. I felt tortured, embarrassed, and conflicted.

As Sammy and I sat at that restaurant and talked about pool, my only interest at the time, I interrupted him.

"I have a problem," I told Sammy. "I have a friend who might have gotten herself into a pickle." I told Sammy what my "friend" had done, how she had let some people talk her into an illegal electronics scheme.

Sammy saw right through my story. He knew that my "friend" was me, and our conversation quickly turned very serious, and very personal. I told Sammy, in my heart, I knew it was wrong, but I didn't know what to do.

It was a gamble. The money was easy, but there was the risk of getting caught. And backing out seemed like a bigger risk, with Jake's shadow hovering.

Sammy paused for a moment, and then he said, "I can't tell you what to do. Only you can make that decision."

I'll never forget what Sammy said next. He asked me who the two most important people in my life were. That answer was easy. It was my mother and my grandfather, who had died when I was 21 years old.

At that dinner table, our food barely touched, Sammy told me to close my eyes and imagine that I was in a room alone with only cold walls, dripping water, and steel bars all around me.

"You're just standing there in a cold and lonely jail cell. Now, imagine opening your eyes, and waking up with your mother and your grandfather on the other side of the bars. Look at their faces," Sammy said. "Can you picture their faces as they are there to pick you up from jail, to try to bail you out, except it's too far, you're in too deep."

Sammy's words struck me like a bolt of lightning. I sat there, and I pictured looking up at my grandfather and my mom, their disappointment, their sadness. I couldn't bear the thought of how they would feel about me. If I landed in jail, that would destroy them.

No, I told Sammy, that can't happen.

"It's only a matter of time," Sammy said, staring deep into my eyes. "Is that look on your mother's face when she finds out what you've done worth the risk of getting this money?"

In that instant, Sammy made the decision for me. I was done with Jake the Snake, no matter the price.

Nearly 15 years later, I finally got to tell Sammy how thankful I was for what he had done for me, wrangling me away from Jake's deceitful scheme. I was at a pro event in 2005 when I ran into Sammy. I did a double take. Was this really him?

"Sammy, is that you?" I asked him. It was. It was Sammy Kong, now much older, much more frail, and still so kind.

I looked at Sammy in that moment and I told him what an incredible impact he'd had on me. I told him I knew my life could have, probably would have, turned out very differently if I had followed my illegal path. I owed a lot to him for my incredible billiards career.

Sammy smiled and he told me thank you, but then he did something completely unexpected. He had a gift for me.

In 2001, I had written a book, *The Black Widow's Guide to Killer Pool.* My book had not been well promoted because, just as it was coming out, I was going through a series of surgeries on my neck, back, and shoulder. I never went on a book tour, and most people, to be honest, didn't even know I had written a book. That always made me really sad.

But Sammy had taken my book, had it leather bound and, inside, he had written me a heartfelt, personal message. Sammy had believed in me, even when I didn't believe in myself.

I certainly didn't believe in myself the morning after I met Sammy for that dinner where he helped me make my decision to give up the gig with Jake the Snake. When it was time for me to report to Jake a few days later for my second illegal purchase, I never showed up.

I nervously went back to Chelsea Billiards to practice the next day, and I went back the next day, and week after week. I was always worried I would see Jake there, and that he would be angry. I was always worried Jake would tell people what I had done.

But Jake wasn't there, and I breathed a sigh of relief. Three weeks passed, then five weeks passed, then eight weeks passed, and I thought maybe I would never see him again.

Then one day, months after I stole electronics from Macy's, I saw Jake across the pool hall.

I took a deep breath, looked at him, and said, "Jake, I can't do it anymore. And man, I promise you, I will never say anything to anyone. I will never take that chance. I just want to play pool."

I stood there, 19 years old, quivering and horrified as Jake took a long, hard look at me. He was quiet as he stared at me, and I was scared to death, scared this was going to ruin my pool career. But then, after what seemed like hours, Jake said one incredible word to me: "Alright."

Jake the Snake was releasing me from his illegal web.

When I ran into Jake after that, he acted as if nothing had ever happened. There were no evil words. There were no threats. I saw Jake a few more times after that, and our exchanges were always just a nod.

After he enlisted me in his plot, Jake was never a regular at Chelsea Billiards like he had been before. Maybe Jake the Snake was as scared of me as I was of him.

Either way, what I did with Jake sent me on a mission to become better, not just in life, but in pool.

In my second big tournament as an amateur, I came in third out of 96 women. It was a magical moment. It was like something you see in a movie. I was like the Hickory Huskers basketball team from the movie *Hoosiers*.

I knew then I was worth more than what Jake the Snake thought I was worth. Inside my tiny, cramped apartment, I hung Post-It notes with motivational words. *You can be great. Hard work pays off. You can overcome. You will succeed.*

Very soon, those words became reality when, in what the billiards industry has called a sensational, meteoric rise, my hard work really did pay off.

I became the No. 1 pool player in the world.

CHAPTER 10

AN IMPROBABLE WHIRLWIND RISE TO NO. 1

PEOPLE HAVE CALLED ME an overnight billiards sensation. They have called my rise to becoming the No. 1 women's pool player in the world meteoric, like an arrow soaring straight up into the sky at lightning speed.

It did not feel meteoric to me. From the time I picked up a cue to the time I became a pro to the time I became No. 1, I put in millions of hours of practice—at least it felt like millions of hours of practice. It felt very, very slow to me.

Sometimes, it seemed as if I was pushing on the gas at full speed, but the brakes were permanently stuck on. I would go home alone to my apartment at night and wonder what in the hell was taking me so long.

What was wrong with me? Why was I learning so slowly? Why did I keep missing so many easy shots so carelessly? How long was it going to take to become the best?

Looking back now, 30 years later, I know becoming a pro by the age of 21, three years after walking into Chelsea Billiards, and becoming No. 1 in the world by the age of 23 was insanely fast. If I think about it logically, I know that.

But I put so much blood, sweat, and tears into my rise to the top, that it didn't feel fast at all.

Looking back, I can see so many things that gave me an edge to rise so quickly. And one of those was the gambling at Chelsea Billiards. That pool club went from a hot scene for yuppies and businessmen when it opened to *the place* to go for gambling within a year or two.

And there I was, gambling right along with the best of them into the wee hours of the night. It's hard to describe that magical time for me, being in a dark pool hall with all men, men who respected me because when we gambled, I could beat them.

After playing and gambling at the local pool halls and in local tournaments and repeatedly winning, I started playing in regional tournaments. Sometimes, JoAnn Mason or Dawn Hopkins, two of the great women pro players of the time, would come to those tournaments.

The other amateur women players were annoyed by that, and they would gripe about it. They didn't want the pros there, these women who could trounce them. I could never understand what they were thinking, why they were complaining about that. I was always ecstatic to see those great players' names on the roster.

For a $25 entry fee, I got to play a pro. I welcomed that with open arms. I wanted nothing more than to go at those women and beat them.

As I played in those regional tournaments, sometimes getting my ass kicked and sometimes winning, I started realizing I could actually make a career out of this crazy, wonderful game. I could make a career doing what I loved every single day, playing pool.

> "She was quite young, but then she told me and my mom she was winning the local tournaments. She was winning and rising through the ranks very fast and she thought she could do this as a career, and she wanted to do it. I don't remember my mom opposing her. I think my mom was just like, 'Are you sure you can do that?'"
>
> —Doris Lee, Jeanette's sister

To me, it definitely felt like my mother was 100 percent opposed to the idea of me making pocket billiards a career. That was not my parents' American dream. Here I was a young Korean woman, part of a family who wanted nothing more than academic success and life success, who were driven to succeed.

I'm not sure my parents had ever really even heard of the sport of pool. They had definitely not heard of it being something you could make a career out of.

I was so nervous when I went to my parents and told them what I wanted to do. They were not happy. They told me I was wasting my life. I knew I wasn't wasting my life. I was positive I could do this.

But to make a career out of billiards, I needed sponsors. Pool was expensive, and there was no way I could afford the game on my own. I needed to fund my own travel to get to tournaments. I needed to pay for hotels and food. I needed to pay for tournament entry fees, which, at some of the bigger events, were very expensive.

My parents didn't have disposable income and, even if they had, they definitely weren't willing to use it to support my pool ambitions.

At my second pro event, the Willards Open, I met John Lewis, who was a board member of the Billiards Congress of America, the billiards trade organization that governed both amateur and professional pool in America. He watched me battle my way through the tournament to finish third place out of 96 of the best women players in the world. I told him about my dream to go pro and become the best. He suggested I take a trip to the BCA tradeshow and introduce myself to the different billiard companies for sponsorship. When I got home, I got out the yellow pages and found a writer to create a résumé for me with the local news clippings of me that I showed him and a list of all the local and regional tournaments I had won. It cost me $30. I was mostly playing at Amsterdam Billiards Club on the Upper West Side at that point. One of the regulars was Stan Schaffer, a world-renowned photographer that had an incredible portfolio of Hollywood stars and Victoria's Secret models. He was kind enough to invite me to pop in at one of his photo shoots and had their makeup artist do my makeup. He took photos of me that blew me away. I had *never* seen myself look that pretty. I was so happy. I had 8x10s and my résumé printed. I got a couple books at Barnes & Noble on self-promotion, marketing, and self-branding, and off I went. It was terrifying, but I felt I had to do it because day jobs took too much of my time away from pool. I needed to make money. I needed a career.

I was very aggressive. I wanted to establish myself quickly and get financial backing.

Many years later, my mom told me how proud she was of me for taking that initiative. She was proud that I had made my career without anyone helping me.

"Jeanette, you really did it all on your own dime and on your own terms," my mother said to me. "And you made it to No. 1 without having any help at all." Hearing my mother say that was one of the happiest moments of my life. She meant, I went after pool without asking her to fund it or me in any way. Of course I had help every step of the way. At Chelsea, then Amsterdam Billiards Club, La Cue, Royal Billiards, Bayside Billiards, and Howard Beach Billiard Club. There were so many nice people that helped along my journey in one way or another.

As I scratched and clawed my way to secure sponsors, I did the same playing in tournaments.

In the Tri-State area, there was a monthly tournament, which included New York, New Jersey, and Pennsylvania. The tournament was for both women and men, but it was mostly the men who showed up. I loved taking on the men.

And I was okay with losing to the men, too, because I was learning, and there weren't a lot of women willing to get in there and wrestle with the guys. Even in those early days of playing, I was drawing a crowd.

I felt the love from the fans almost from the beginning. I didn't have a name for it then, and I still don't have a name for it now. I guess it was presence, and I don't mean that in a cocky way.

I was simply gaining attention, because I was constantly the only woman playing in the men's tournaments. And playing against the men, I firmly believe, is what catapulted me to the top of the women's game.

> "A lot of her life was spent matching up and gambling against men's players. Jeanette was the equal of many men's players. She couldn't break the rack really hard because of her back. That was the one shot she couldn't have. But she would just smash them. Her offensive game was just so beautiful to watch."
>
> —Don Wardell, Lee's longtime physician and friend

It was at a women's regional tournament in 1991 that I got the break of my career, that big break superstars always talk about. I had been playing in all these different tournaments, in New York City, upstate New York, Pittsburgh, Long Island, and all the way up to Maine and Rhode Island.

I would drive anywhere I could for a tournament that paid big. I was, after all, used to podunk tournaments where the entry fees were $5 or $10, and the payout was, sometimes, only the money you put in. I eventually worked my way up to $25 fees and then $50 fees.

Then I found out about the state championships being held with $75 or $100 entry fees. That was a major investment for me, still a struggling kid.

But whenever I would win prize money, even if it was 30 bucks, it never went toward fancy food or splurges on brand-name fashion clothing or posh spa treatments. I always rolled that money over. That money was what paid for my next tournament.

And in 1991, I had scrounged up enough money to enter the New York State Championship, where I finished in second place. Any normal pool player, at the level I was at, would have been overjoyed with that finish. I was bitterly disappointed.

The winner of that state championship got a free slot to compete in the Women's Professional Billiard Association Nationals, which was, and still is, one of the most prestigious tournaments you can win in pool. It's like making it to the Masters tournament in golf.

I wasn't disappointed for long. The pool gods, for some reason, seemed to be watching over me. The woman who beat me in that New York State Championship unexpectedly dropped out, which meant my second-place finish gave me the slot—my launch into the WPBA tour.

Less than three years after I first picked up a piece of chalk, I joined the WPBA tour, "a remarkably swift ascent for someone with her relative lack of experience," wrote *Sports Illustrated.*

Here I was, a kid from New York, and I was playing in the WPBA National Championships, my first pro tournament ever. It was an amazing, gratifying moment for me. I had finally broken my way into the elite echelon of billiards.

I quickly took the women's tour by storm, winning the WPBA nationals and making it to the finals of the U.S. Open 9-Ball Championship in 1993 to claim the No. 1 ranking.

It was an incredible feeling to clinch that No. 1 spot, to have the other women on the tour finally acknowledge that I wasn't just some pretty face who wore tight, black clothing, and called myself "The Black Widow."

> "She came on hot and heavy, like a bull in a China closet. But the good thing about Jeanette was that she proved it."
>
> —Loree Jon Jones,
> an eight-time world champion
> and one of Lee's biggest rivals

At the 1994 U.S. Open 9-Ball Championship in Chesapeake, Virginia, I took on Ewa Mataya in the final match. I was focused, I wanted that title.

"She played fast and fierce," Mataya said at the time. "She was on fire. All of a sudden, Jeanette was just the one to beat."

I won an unheard-of number of professional titles in the next six years, one title in 1995, two in 1996, four in 1997, 11 in 1999, and 14 in 2000. "Jeanette started going off like gangbusters," said Mike Panozzo, publisher of *Billiards Digest*.

As I started winning big cash, my friend and fellow pool player John Lewis asked me, "What are you going to do with the money?" Of course, I was going to take my winnings and use them to enter more tournaments. That was always my mission: to win and to enter more tournaments.

I'll never forget what John said to me. And he said it firmly: "Jeanette, you need to buy something nice for yourself, something really nice."

At the time, when I was first starting out, tournaments didn't give out trophies, just prize money. There was no physical relic to take home. John told me to take my winnings and use a portion of it to buy myself something to symbolize my victory: a fancy pair of shoes, a designer handbag, or an ornate vase.

"After a while, your whole house will be filled," John told me. "You will be surrounded by your own successes. And that will keep you going."

So that's what I did.

When I won $3,500 in my second pro tournament, placing third out of 96 women, a literal nobody coming out of nowhere, I bought my first pair of leather Stuart Weitzman boots that went four inches above my knees. They cost $580 and they were the most beautiful pair of shoes I had ever seen. Before that, I had never spent more than $70 on shoes.

I still have those thigh-high boots in my closet to this day. They are a sentimental, wonderful memento of my first big win.

From then on, after I won a tournament I would always buy myself one really nice thing, and then stash the rest of the cash away for necessities. I ended up buying myself a lot of nice things, because I kept winning.

When I was beating the other players, it was bad for them, but it was great for me. I had never felt confident about anything in life. But at the pool table, there was no reason for me not to feel confident, and I became a sensation.

When ESPN2 began airing the WPBA tour, my career got a life-altering, landscape-altering, unexpected shot in the arm. Everything changed. Every single thing in my life changed.

Being on ESPN2 provided a major boost to my visibility. The network really liked The Black Widow, and it made me its women's billiards star.

> "To get to Jeanette's rise in the sport, nobody's paying attention unless it's on ESPN. I have been in Wimbledon locker rooms, I've been in NBA locker rooms, where Jeanette's on the air on ESPN2, and those guys are gathered around and they're rooting for her. They were not watching pool. They

> were watching Jeanette. These big stars were watching her because she was a big star, too."
>
> —Tom George, Lee's longtime manager

Some people said those men were watching me because I was beautiful. I believe they were watching me because I was good.

Every professional tournament I have ever entered, from my first match 30 years ago to the one I played in September 2021 after finishing chemo, I have never failed to take home cash. I have never finished out of the money throughout my entire professional career.

That is an unheard-of accomplishment in any sport. It would be like a player on the PGA tour making the cut in every single tournament, except that in the sport of pool, it was even harder. In most tournaments, the money only went to the top eight players. Some bigger events would pay out up to 10th, or 12th, or maybe 16th place.

Because of my lifetime streak of always taking home money, some of the women on the tour thought I was full of myself, but I wasn't. I was simply confident because I was winning.

> "I don't think it was swagger [Jeanette had]. I think it just makes people mad when you have this belief in yourself and then you do exactly what you say you're going to do."
>
> —Jennifer Barretta,
> a top women's player and competitor
> of Lee's, *Jeanette Lee Vs.*

I saw the table differently than most players saw the table. I saw the angles and geometry. When I became No. 1, people would ask me how many balls I could see ahead. To be honest, sometimes it was the whole rack. I could see 15 shots ahead. I could see the whole table in an uncanny way.

When I was playing pool at an elite level, I listened to a lot of mental imagery tapes. I would close my eyes and I would imagine myself draining every single shot into the pocket, no matter how tough that shot was.

I would make cassette tapes where I recorded encouraging messages to myself. "I'm strong. I'm confident. I rise to any opportunity. I step up to the challenge. I'm decisive. I stalk the table like a panther. I'm committed to every shot."

On the other side of the tape I would remind myself what it took physically. "Keep a loose grip throughout the swing. Be a pendulum. Elbow stays up in the air. Keep a firm bridge. Stay down and follow through. Watch alignment. Stay balanced."

Whenever I was in the car or working out or doing anything other than playing pool, I would listen to those tapes over and over again.

Inside my apartment in L.A., I had tiny little reminders all over. I would take little, yellow Post-It notes with words of affirmation written on them and I would plaster them all over the place. I would stick them to my bathroom mirror, on the refrigerator door, on the microwave, and on my bedroom nightstand. I had them taped to the dashboard of my car and written in notebooks that I carried inside my purse.

I was dead serious about becoming the best pool player in the world. Throughout my career, I won every major title in billiards, more than 30 national and international titles, including a gold medal at the 2001 World Games in Akita, Japan.

I was the WPBA Sportsperson of the Year, earned Player of the Year honors from both *Billiards Digest* and *Pool & Billiard Magazine*, was honored with the 2001 BBIA Industry Service Award, was the 2004 International Trick Shot champion, and took home back-to-back Empress Cup titles in 2008 and 2009.

My proudest moments came as I was inducted into three different halls of fame, the Billiard Congress of America and WPBA Hall of Fame in 2013, and the Asian Hall of Fame in 2015, which wasn't just about sports. It was about stardom.

Those hall of fame ceremonies always brought back memories of how I had gotten to that elite space. How hard I had fought, not just at the pool table, but in life.

There was, after all, always the scoliosis that was trying to take me down, the brutal back pain that plagued my body. And there was my family life, my parents who didn't understand my quest to be a billiards world champion.

> "I did not like Jeanette being out so late, her coming home at 3:00 and 4:00 AM. All the men she was around? I worried so much about her."
>
> —Sonja Lee, Jeanette's mother

I don't blame her one bit. The older I get, and as a mother of three teenage daughters myself, the worse I feel about the stress and agony I put my mom through. At the time, though, none of that mattered to me, and what my parents didn't give me in support as I rose to the top of my game, I got from the men at the pool rooms.

Chelsea Billiards soon became known as the best place to get action in New York City. Pros and hustlers invaded the club, and being around that caliber of players had a huge impact on me. It kept me hungry to get better, and it gave me an idea of how great the game of pool could be played.

Chelsea may have been the first pool hall I walked into, but there were other pool rooms that made indelible marks on my career.

There was Amsterdam Billiards Club, which was founded in 1989 in Manhattan by comedian David Brenner and two brothers, Greg and Ethan Hunt. Brenner's comedian friends, Jerry Seinfeld and Richard Lewis, would play pool there, and they would sit in the front row to watch the pro events the club hosted.

Amsterdam's owners knew how to attract the yuppies from the Upper West Side. Whenever a really good player showed up they would be added to the pro list and get free table time. Soon, I was added to that list, and instead of Chelsea I started going to Amsterdam to play for free.

I got my first and only paid pool lesson at the club, when Greg Hunt paid his house pro, Abe Rosen, $30 to shower me with his billiards knowledge. Greg was always my biggest advocate, helping in any way he could to advance my career.

To make extra money, I waitressed at Amsterdam, and it was around that time I started playing seriously in all the local tournaments. Greg helped me pay for entry fees as the club sponsored me. I soon became one of the best in New York City, outside of the top pros, Billie Billing, Fran Crimi, and JoAnn Mason.

It was at Amsterdam that I set the current women's world record of 152 consecutive balls in straight pool.

Soon, I started making my way to other pool halls to practice. There was Elite Billiards, which is where I met my longtime mentor, Gene Nagy. When it shut down, Gene and I moved to La Cue Billiards. We played countless games there. Soon, Howard Beach Billiard Club sponsored me for my first pro event, then my second pro event, and then my third pro event.

When I finally made it to the No. 1 player in the world, I couldn't believe I had gotten there. I remember thinking, "This is all I had to do?" I thought it should have been harder. I thought, to be the top-ranked woman, I should have been a better player.

As the media came calling to do articles and broadcasts on me at all those different pool halls, they would always ask me about my rise. "How did you get here, Jeanette?" "What is your secret?" "Who taught you how to play?"

That last question always irked me.

I have been around so many pro men's pool players getting interviewed, and when they're asked who taught them the game, most of them say nobody. They were self-taught. The interviewer usually says, "Oh, wow," and moves on.

When I would tell reporters that I was self-taught, they would say, "No, no, no, somebody had to teach you how to play."

No. Nobody *taught* me how to play. I *watched* the men play, and I wanted to imitate them. I watched those men as I played them. I watched so intently that I would go home at night and dream about the shots they were taking.

And one of those men who I watched, probably more than any player, was my billiards mentor Gene Nagy. He taught me just about everything I know.

He was magical, otherworldly, and he was a lost soul, just like I had been.

CHAPTER 11

AN UNLIKELY FRIENDSHIP WITH A BILLIARDS MANIAC

BY THE TIME I MET GENE NAGY, he was a lonely, gruff, bushy-bearded man who could usually be found riding his bicycle through the streets of New York City. Gene never went anywhere by car. He was afraid of automobiles, though he never really could explain why.

Gene was a broken man when I met him, a former billiards superstar who had shined the brightest when he was high on drugs. Now, he wore suspenders over short-sleeved shirts with baggy jeans, black tennis shoes, and a bag strung across his shoulder, biking to the only place he ever went.

A pool hall.

When I met Gene, he was no longer a maniacal, ranting, world champion at the table. He was a shell of who he once was, now just a guy who played alone or with a couple of the younger regulars, quietly in the corner.

At the height of his career, Gene had been a legendary straight-pool competitor, known in New York City in the late 1960s and early '70s as maybe the greatest player on the scene. But before that, he was great at something else. He was an elite, accomplished musician.

Gene started playing the trumpet at the age of 12 and attended the Juilliard School of Music at 17. He was a musical genius who performed at Carnegie Hall.

By the time I met Gene in the early '90s, he was mysterious, captivating, dark, kind of handsome, and old enough to be my dad. I was 19, just starting my career. Gene was in his early forties. It just so happened a friend of mine was a friend of Gene's, and he thought we should meet. Maybe Gene could help me with my game.

I met Gene at a pool hall in New York City called Elite Billiards. I was so scared, so intimidated. I didn't know what to say. I got a set of balls and started playing on a table near his, playing the best pool I could play, hoping he'd notice and it would spark some interest. I'm not sure he even noticed I was in the room. Finally, my friend Vinny introduced me and asked if he would play a few games with me.

I had heard the stories about Gene Nagy, one of the greatest billiards players to ever hail from New York, who was now a loner who never seemed to smile, and who everyone was scared to talk to.

But when I met Gene for the first time, he put me at ease. He was this gentle soul wearing a tough exterior to keep everyone from seeing the good stuff. But I saw it. I saw all the good in gentle Gene.

Everything I know about billiards—and a lot about life—I learned from Gene. He was my coach, my mentor, my friend, a father figure. He was my everything.

Eventually, Elite closed down and Gene Nagy, Bob Watson, Jimmy, Vinny, and a couple other guys started hanging out at La Cue Billiards and Cafe in Maspeth, Queens. I, of course, followed. After spending years playing regulars at Chelsea Billiards, and then

Amsterdam Billiards, I had the opportunity to play one of the greatest players that ever lived, completely for free. He never charged me to play straight pool with him, and the few young regulars that used to take turns playing him all stepped aside so that I could have him to myself—playing pool, I mean. I'm so thankful for that. I didn't really think about it at the time. Mike and Bernie, the owners, were retired police officers and they shared our love of the game. They were kind enough to give us both free table time whenever we played there.

I would show up to the pool hall at 10:00 AM and Gene would be there next to his bike on the sidewalk waiting for me. The tables didn't open until 11:00 AM, so Gene and I would grab a cup of coffee in the cafe and he'd share pool stories of his past. He also said to forget having boyfriends and drugs because romance ruins your pool game and drugs ruin your life.

When the doors opened, we would walk to the table and our talking would come to an abrupt end. We were in the zone. We were focused. We would play game after game after game, until we were forced out of the hall as the lights turned off at 3:00 AM. Depending on which manager was closing that night, sometimes they'd lock all the doors and turn all the outdoor lights off, and four or five of us would keep playing all night until we'd get breakfast together. I'd go home, get as little sleep as I could bear, and race back to La Cue to do it all over again. I miss those days.

Gene and I did that every single day, usually for at least 15 hours, with small breaks in-between for my back pain, until I left New York to chase my professional career. Gene never charged me a dime for those hours of play, for those thousands of hours of wisdom a pool icon gave me, teaching me his secrets, and never once trying to beat me.

The entire time I played with Gene, even after I was a pro, we never kept score. Gene never played a race. He just played. There was no other option. I would have never dared ask Gene, "Hey, would you like to play a set or race to five games, best of seven?"

For Gene, this wasn't about winning or losing. This was about playing for the love of the game. To grow our knowledge and improve our skills. We just played, no pressure. It sounds like that would have been monotonous, boring, and mind-numbing, but it wasn't. Not when you were playing with Gene Nagy.

He made these shots that were unbelievable. He made shots that, had TikTok been around back then, would have gone viral. Gene never seemed too amazed by his own ability. But he always seemed to know that he could control a table. He was a badass to me. I fell in love with the way Gene played pool.

Because Gene never kept score, I was given the freedom to try anything. I was constantly finding out what worked and what didn't work. I would watch him go for shots, and I would stop him and ask, "Wait. What are you trying to do?"

Gene would just blow my mind, calling these insane shots. I would call insane shots, too. I would try low-percentage shots, just to see if it was possible, and, because of that, my knowledge kept increasing. I knew what was possible because I didn't worry about the score and just went for it.

I studied how the cue ball trickled off the other balls, how the balls danced, how one tiny knock could send a ball in a direction you didn't expect. Gene and I shared a love of the intricacies of straight pool, a game that was more common to our billiard forefathers. It's the same game that Jackie Gleason and Paul Newman played in *The Hustler*. It was also played in the 55th episode of *The Twilight Zone*. It was a love, and a sickness. An obsession. My time playing with him was like being stuck in a lab with a mad scientist. And it was wonderful.

Gene used to tell me that during his days as a pro, he would drive himself into madness.

> "I was driven in those days like there was an evil spirit inside me. I thought I could train myself to be a machine and play perfect pool all the time. I wanted to do the impossible, to never miss. I know now that that was crazy."
>
> —Gene Nagy, *Newsday*, August 1992

As I honed my skills, Gene took me under his wings, and I drank in everything he told me, everything he did. It was like a hyper focus when I watched him.

I know this might sound conceited, and I don't mean it in a conceited way, but I notice things that most people don't notice. I just do. It's not something I can brag about. I think it's something I was born with.

When I watched Nagy, I took in so much more than him dropping balls in the pocket. I watched his breathing, his tempo, his stance, his stroke, his fundamentals, his choices. He taught me a true, pure, strategic, geometrical love of the game.

And he taught me that I could be great. Gene had this calm, relentless faith in me. He really believed that I could become the best woman player ever.

I know how lucky I was to get to learn from Gene, to have him at my disposal. I had a very high-level competitor playing with me every day in those early years. Not many people get that.

On some evenings, after a day of soaking in everything I could from Gene, I would leave him at 6:00 PM to play in local, weekly tournaments at other pool halls. Each week, I noticed how much better I was playing in those tournaments. I knew Gene was to thank for that.

But, in those early days, I didn't win all those tournaments, and that frustrated me. I hated losing. I would come back home all pissed off. As I fell asleep, I would think about the shot I missed that cost me the match.

I would get up the next day, go to the pool hall, and shoot that shot 400 times. It was always 400 times. Sometimes, I felt like I was punishing myself for missing the shot. I wasn't. I was trying to get better. I always wanted to take any weakness I had and turn it into a weapon.

Gene never came to my tournaments. The entire time I knew him, he only went to one place, to a pool hall. I was never hurt that Gene didn't come to watch me play.

I knew the first time I met Gene that he was different. He was guarded, he was closed off from most of the world. But somehow, he was a man that found a way to dig deep into his shattered soul and love me.

When Gene came into my life, I was a shattered soul, too, who had suffered a lot of disappointments. I was insecure and I wasn't sure anyone could love me.

It was comforting to show up to the pool hall and have Gene waiting there for me, every single day. Gene changed my entire view on life. He gave me an optimism that I didn't have before. He taught me so much.

I was always hyper competitive. But when I played with Gene, I learned not to worry about the score and to love the beauty of billiards. Gene made me a student of the game. He taught me to never get too high on myself, thinking I knew too much. He stressed that even the greatest pool player should always believe they could learn something new.

The hallmark of any good player is her ability to run over 100 balls in straight pool. Gene knew this, so once I got good enough to run 80 or 90 balls, we started keeping track of my runs. When I first broke 100 by running 122 consecutive balls, we celebrated like crazy. Then, the very next inning, Gene ran 238 balls. Now *that's* a pool lesson.

I know some of my opponents would say I didn't have humility. They thought I was cocky. But I always knew I could be better, because Gene had taught me that.

Gene was always my biggest advocate, trying to help me become a better, happier, more fulfilled version of myself. He also instilled in me the value of staying away from drugs and how it could wreck your life. He was my supporter, my ally, and my encouragement. He kept my soul alive, and, at the table, he always kept me hungry for the game.

I never took it for granted, getting to play with Gene. I was honored he was there by my side. Gene was, after all, a world champion.

He was a neurotic world champion who, during the height of his career, turned the world of pool upside down with his wild antics and unexplainable behavior. As Gene rose to billiards fame, there were times he felt obsessed, he once said, almost as if he were going mad.

Just about anyone who crossed paths with Gene, his competitors, his fans, and the media, called him "Crazy Gene." At the height of his career, he was known as much for his erratic tirades and self-destructive behavior as he was for his genius at pool playing.

Gene was a perfectionist who hated that he couldn't be perfect.

"He'd shoot like God one moment and act like a maniac the next," Pete Margo, a former top player, told *Newsday* in 1992. "When things didn't go Gene's way, he was capable of almost anything."

As he battled in matches, Gene would smash custom-made cues into pieces, tear up wads of cash, throw balls across the pool hall, and put out cigarettes on the back of his hand. One match, Gene charged the wall headfirst at full speed.

> "I can laugh at it now, but at the time it wasn't funny. The stress caused by my own imperfection was killing me. I just couldn't accept being imperfect."
>
> —Gene Nagy, *Newsday*, August 1992

So Gene turned to drugs. The first time he took amphetamine, he was 22 years old. Gene was playing at a tournament in Georgia and he was missing every single shot. Some guy, a guy Gene didn't know, walked up to him after the match and said, "You want some heart, kid? Here."

That guy handed Gene two pills. They were interesting looking pills; clear-and-green capsules with white "beads" inside. And because of their holiday color scheme they were known as "Christmas trees." They were also known as Dexamyl Spansule.

The next morning, Gene ate those two Christmas trees for breakfast, went to the tournament, and didn't miss a shot.

In that moment, Gene was hooked. He started using drugs as he became a world champion. The uppers made him alert. Everything was crystal clear as he played. Gene once said the drugs made him so intense he could see the tiny fibers of the green felt on the table.

During tournaments, the rumor among his opponents was that if Gene went to the bathroom during a match, you couldn't beat him.

Gene never tried to hide that he popped pills like popcorn. He would get so high, or low, that he would foam at the mouth as he played. Sometimes, he didn't know where he was.

> "Gene wasn't shy about telling the whole world about it. He'd say, 'I'm just gonna pop these Black Beauties and run out all night.' We'd just look at each other cross-eyed in disbelief."
>
> —Pete Margo,
> former top pool player, *Newsday*, August 1992

Gene called it "being on the juice." He used different drugs, depending on what game he was playing. He took speed for the rapid, intense action of 9-ball, and he took tranquilizers for the slower pace of straight pool.

On the juice, Gene became one of the best, most feared, players on the circuit. Gene's lifetime personal high run of 430 is topped officially only by Thomas Engert, John Schmidt, Jayson Shaw, Min-Wai Chin, and Willie Mosconi, according to *Billiards Digest*. He is also known for running 150 and out in the 1973 World Straight Pool Open against Allen Hopkins.

"It was the finest I had ever seen balls taken from the table," Willie Mosconi, widely considered one of the greatest pool players of all time, said of Gene's performance.

> "Gene Nagy, that man was born to play this game."
>
> —Luther Lassiter,
> renowned American pool player,
> who won six world billiards championships

But by the late 1970s, when Gene was only in his early thirties, he retired from competition. He was a world champion who quietly, with no fanfare, suddenly disappeared.

As the years passed, many wondered what had become of Gene Nagy. He wasn't playing on the elite circuit. He was just playing in local halls, mentoring up-and-coming players like me.

I knew why Gene had stepped away from the pro game. Gene was always afraid of the pressure. He couldn't take the heat. He had bookies who would stuff him full of speed and make him feel like he was on top of the world.

And when Gene was on top of the world, no one could beat him. He felt free and uninhibited. But when he quit the drugs, he couldn't play in high-level competition. The nerves overtook him, and he literally just fell apart.

He turned to a life of everyday, casual, behind-the-scenes billiards, coaching and mentoring young players. I'm not sure Gene ever had any idea how thankful I was for that.

Gene was the closest thing to the kind of father I had always wanted, the kind of man I could go to for advice. I called him my pool dad. There were so many days and nights I'd get into an argument with my mom that ended in her telling me I was wasting my life.

I would go to the pool hall; I would turn to Gene. I would tell him my concerns that my mom was disappointed in me. He would shrug his shoulders and mumble, "Don't worry, Jeanette, you're going to be a star, and your mother will see that you're working hard. It will all work out in the end. Just keep doing what you are doing and then she'll see."

Gene would tell me that my mother loved me and that she was just worried about me, that she couldn't understand what I was doing, playing pool. He told me that one day she would understand.

With tears in my eyes, I would play Gene all day and night and, when I played, my mother and everything else that was bothering me would dissipate. That's why I loved pool so much. It took away all the voices of self-doubt and self-criticism, the feelings of ineptness and deficiency.

After I went on the pro tour and, as the years passed, I didn't get to see Gene as much as I wanted to. I was on the West Coast and he was in New York. But as my pool career forged ahead, Gene and I always remained close. We didn't write, but I visited him every year on every trip to New York to see my family or for business except in 2005. It was such a busy year and the two trips I made to New York that year were very short ones, so I didn't go see him. God I wish I did.

But in the summer of 2006, I found out that Gene was keeping a secret from me. He was very sick. His emphysema and lung cancer had taken a turn for the worse. He was gravely ill with not much time left.

Gene had sworn everyone who knew me to secrecy, to not tell me how sick he was. He knew I would put my career on hold and come to New York to take care of him until he died. He didn't want me to do that. He always put my career ahead of anything else.

As Gene's final days were imminent, my friend and fellow pool player, Bob Watson, called me and told me that if I wanted to see Gene alive, I should go soon. I was absolutely devastated.

I was at the *ESPYs* in Los Angeles, getting ready to work the red carpet for ESPN, holding a microphone and interviewing superstar athletes as they walked into the Kodak Theatre. I decided when I got home Monday, I would book a one-way plane ticket to New York and stay as long as Gene needed me. Stay with him until the end.

But when I got on the red carpet, all I could think about was Gene. My heart was aching, I felt so sad and so guilty that I was at a glitzy awards show among sports stardom and Gene, the man who had gotten me on that red carpet, was dying in a hospital.

I called my husband, George, and told him I wouldn't be coming home from the *ESPYs* Monday. After it was over, I would fly straight to New York. But then, as I got to the curtain call that night, waiting to take my seat, something magical happened.

As I stood by the curtains, Reggie Bush walked up to me. He was smiling from ear to ear. "Hey, it's Reggie," he said to me. I had no idea who he was. I had no idea he was the 2005 Heisman Trophy winner, and I had no idea he was the kid I'd met on an airplane years before.

When Reggie was nine years old, I was seated next to him and his dad on a flight to San Diego. Reggie and I sat next to each other and talked the entire flight. He told me he loved football. I gave him an autograph, but I also asked him to send me a school photo of him and to sign it, because, I told him, I knew he would be famous one day too.

And there Reggie was, in 2006, behind the curtains with me at the *ESPYs*, telling me how I had motivated him and how I had inspired him through the years to never give up, and to always be kind to the fans. It was an incredible moment, a joyful moment, and it was a full circle moment.

After Reggie walked away, I knew what I had to do. I couldn't stay for the *ESPYs*. I had to leave. I had to catch the red eye now. I had to get to Gene, the man who had inspired me. I had to get to his hospital bed. My ESPN bosses were wonderful to me. "Go, Jeanette. Go see Gene," they told me.

I left the *ESPYs* that night and I arrived at Gene's bedside early the next morning. He was in a medically induced coma to help with the intense pain. I tried to talk to him, but the nurses told me he wouldn't be able to hear me.

I took Gene's hand anyway, and I told him I loved him. I told him I was so sorry I hadn't been there sooner. I told him I felt guilty for that, and I told him what he had meant to me. Just then, Gene squeezed my hand.

I jumped up. I was startled, and I was overjoyed. Gene hadn't made a voluntary movement in weeks. I told the nurses that Gene had squeezed my hand, with newfound hope that maybe he would be okay. The nurses assured me that it was just a random movement, that it didn't mean anything.

But as the nurses talked, Gene gripped my hand again and again. He was clenching me.

I truly believe, in those moments, that Gene was telling me he was there, and that he knew I was there. He had heard the words I said to him.

I crawled up into Gene's hospital bed, crying, and I laid with him, holding him, and comforting him. He died in my arms 20 minutes later, on July 13, 2006, at the age of 59. Gene and my biological father, John, died the same year, both in my arms. I had to do the funeral arrangements and eulogy for both of them. It was very sad.

As I said goodbye and walked away from his hospital bed, all those memories of the man who had launched my career came rushing back to me. Where would I have been without Gene Nagy?

I knew, without him, I never would have become The Black Widow.

CHAPTER 12

LEATHER AND LACE: EMERGING AS THE BLACK WIDOW

IT WAS NOT MY IDEA to be called "The Black Widow." It was not my idea to become the human incarnate of a venomous, evil creature with dangerously sharp fangs who murders her lovers after the mating is done.

Why would anyone want to be named after a black widow spider? I hated spiders. I was horrified of spiders.

At one tournament, during the height of my fame in the 1990s, a fan came up to give me a gift. It was, perhaps, the most unusual, yet the most fitting gift I have ever received.

It was a female black widow spider in a cage; an actual real, living, moving, poisonous black widow spider. The thought of that spider inches away from me all those years ago still makes me sick to my stomach.

But I was always polite to fans, so I graciously accepted the creepy, crawling gift and I promptly went home and put the terrarium outside on my balcony in L.A. There was no way I was keeping that thing inside my house.

I was scared that the spider might somehow escape in the middle of the night and crawl onto my bed. I knew if that happened, I would keel over in horror right on the spot.

I kept that little demon on the balcony outside for a few days, until I realized this spider was getting plumper by the hour. My black widow was very pregnant and, if I couldn't handle one spider, how could I handle the 1,000 tiny arachnids—200 in each of her five sacks—that she was about to give birth to?

As I lugged the cage to my car, I told my black widow that I was sorry. I drove her miles away, and I set that spider free in the open country. Don't hate me for what I did. I had my reasons, and they were very good reasons, in my humble opinion.

The black widow spider is a fierce creature, especially the female, whose body is much larger than her male counterpart, and who is always on a mission to kill. The female black widow is chubby and shiny with a red hourglass shape on her abdomen. Her bite contains venom 15 times stronger than a rattlesnake's.

The black widow thrives on biting her prey, eating them alive, and then spitting them out. She is ruthless and evil.

I hated the idea of being nicknamed "The Black Widow."

I had always considered myself sweet. I always had intense empathy for people, almost as if I could feel exactly what others were feeling. I never judged or looked down on anyone. I definitely never thought I was better than anyone else.

I just wanted people to be happy and at peace. I didn't want to hurt them, and I certainly didn't want to eat them alive.

But late one night as the lights were turning off at the Howard Beach Billiard Club in Queens, I unwillingly became The Black Widow.

I had been practicing at Howard Beach, the first million-dollar pool hall to open in the United States, and the club's owner, Gabe

Vigorito, had been watching me. As he came in to lock up one night, I was still there, of course. I could never get enough of the game.

As I headed toward the door to leave, Gabe called me to him, sitting at a table with a cigar in his left hand and an espresso in his right. He stared deep into my eyes, and he said: "Jeanette, you are going to be a champion, and champions need a nickname. I've got the perfect nickname for you—'The Black Widow.'"

No.

No way.

I hated that name. I despised that Gabe or anyone else would ever look at me as a wicked spider. I asked him that night, "How in the world could I remind you of a black widow? I'm super nice. I'm sweet. I'm polite. I don't have a venomous bone in my body."

Gabe insisted the nickname was perfect. "I remember the first day I saw you," he said. "You were smiling at your friends, you were grabbing your cue, talking and laughing, and then boom, you got to the table, and everything changed. You wanted to kill."

A few days after that conversation, in which I did not agree to be called "The Black Widow," I walked into the Howard Beach club. Propped up on every table were brochures. They had a photo of me on the front with the words: "Come play pool with The Black Widow. She really knows how to break balls."

Mortified, I called Gabe immediately, in a fit of panic, and I screeched, "What are you doing? You can't do that." I had agreed to teach lessons at the club, but I had not agreed to teach them as The Black Widow. I pleaded with Gabe to change how he promoted me. I told him no one would understand that name.

"Trust me, they'll understand," he said. "The minute they get to know you, they'll understand."

Gabe went on and on about the first time he watched me play, how I was "a pretty young thing and so sweet." But when I chalked the cue and got down to shoot, my whole persona changed.

> "Jeanette reminded me of a black widow because she would lure her opponents to the table and eat them alive."
>
> —Gabe Vigorito,
> owner of Howard Beach Billiard Club

No matter how I tried to persuade Gabe to give me a different nickname, he wasn't backing down from calling me The Black Widow. He had already printed the brochures, he told me. It was too late.

To be honest, I owe a lot of what I've accomplished in the world of billiards to Gabe, not only for the pool knowledge he gave me, but for The Black Widow persona he created that eventually sucked fans into its web, and caught on like wildfire.

Gabe was persistent and relentless in his quest to make sure I was known as "The Black Widow," and he didn't stop short of bribes.

When I won a spot to play in the WPBA nationals as a rookie in 1991, I was thrilled and then I was devastated. I couldn't afford the trip. The slot only covered the $250 entry fee. It didn't include airfare, a hotel, a rental car, or anything else.

I had never been on an airplane in my life. I didn't know how to book a flight, and I had no clothes to wear that satisfied the tournament's dress code.

And I had no one to turn to. There was no way I could ask my mother for help. We weren't in a good place in our relationship. She couldn't understand why I was so insistent on this outlandish pool obsession.

I was 20 years old, supporting myself, nothing more than a struggling artist with a cue stick, with nothing stashed away in my savings account. I was spending every penny I had for table time and tournament entry fees.

Gabe was my savior. He told me he would cover all my expenses for the WPBA Nationals and give me $500 for a new wardrobe on one condition: everything I bought had to be black.

I raced to the mall and spent the $500. Every single piece I bought was black, from dresses to shoes to dress slacks to earrings to tops. My transformation began. (Though, I should point out that I only bought black dress clothes. I didn't incorporate black leather for a couple years, and I've never bought lacy tops. I gradually became more comfortable with my nickname, but not at first.)

To be honest, becoming The Black Widow was easy for me. It wasn't really that big of a transformation.

I started wearing black when I was 12 and, by the time I was a rebellious runaway teen, my entire wardrobe was edgy. I chopped off my hair, wore military garb and draped bandannas around my neck. My closet was filled with graphic rock 'n' roll T-shirts. My look was dark, and I liked that.

But as I became The Black Widow, I took dark, edgy clothing to a whole new level. I became a fashion icon, even though I never thought of myself that way.

I was blown away when *Vogue* magazine came in 2023 to do a fashion piece on me titled, "The Black Widow, a Pool Legend Reflects on Her Sexy, Boundary-Pushing Style."

> "Lee could often be seen in netted black blouses, leather bustiers, a range of halter tops that emphasized cleavage and revealed just enough of her back to be seen through her waist-length, lustrous black hair. She wore leather trousers, palazzo pants, a variety of black cocktail dresses, and her signature Black Widow billiard glove that covered one half of her hand, exposing a large diamond ring on a perfectly manicured finger."
>
> —Scarlett Newman, *Vogue*, June 2023

That black glove was definitely my signature. Most pool players, especially the women, didn't wear a glove, and I only started wearing it by pure chance.

In the beginning, when I was playing a lot of pool, I just started getting invited to a lot of parties. One night, I was at yet another party, and it was really lame. "Hey, let's sneak out of here and go play," I said to a few friends.

When we got to the billiards club, I still had on the slinky, black dress I'd worn to the party, which included gloves that went all the way up to my armpits. They were skintight and a pain in the butt to get on.

Instead of taking the gloves off, I left them on as I played that night. I loved the feel of the cue, and I loved that I played really well wearing the gloves. When I went back to the pool room the next day, I cut the glove off at the wrist and wore it on my left hand. I started playing every day with that five-fingered silk glove.

I needed to find a different version of the glove and, very soon, I did.

I was at a tournament at the Golden Cue in Queens, one of the oldest pool rooms in New York, when I noticed a player named Danny Barouty wearing a Sure Shot glove, and my mind was blown. Here was this man who was running balls all over the table, wearing a glove, and he was so good.

After his match, I went up to Danny and asked him about the glove. He took me to an old glass case inside the Golden Cue that had chalk, tattered tips, and four black gloves inside. I grabbed one of those gloves and my signature look was born.

The Sir Joseph glove fit well, performed well, and I use their gloves to this day. They were one of my very first sponsors and eventually even added my Black Widow spider to it, so I could sign them and give them to special fans.

I had my black glove and I had black stiletto heels, and my swagger followed. But the swagger was all fake. It wasn't really me.

Jeanette Lee could never have pulled off this look, this persona of The Black Widow. I was still extremely insecure, still that 13-year-old girl wearing a clunky brace, despite the world telling me I was an exotic beauty.

But when I was at the table, I didn't feel like the insecure Jeanette. I felt like a different, braver version of myself, comfortable in my own skin.

I made my debut as The Black Widow at that tournament where Gabe paid for my expenses and made me promise to use the nickname. *New York Times Magazine* was there at the WPBA nationals doing a story on the rise of women's pool, featuring the No. 1 player at the time, Ewa Mataya.

Ewa was the focus of the article, but the writer was looking for other stories to tell, including one about a player from New York City. That reporter found me, a rookie hailing from Brooklyn, playing in my first pro tournament. She asked if I had a nickname. I told her that most people just call me Jeanette.

Then I remembered Gabe, the man who had gotten me to this tournament where I was being interviewed by *New York Times Magazine.*

"Wait," I said to the reporter. "There are some guys at my pool hall that call me 'The Black Widow.'"

The writer smiled. She liked that nickname, and her magazine loved that nickname even more. I became a story in one of the most popular publications in the country, describing me as "a bad Bond girl with a vampish appearance."

And for the first time, the world heard about The Black Widow of pool.

I became America's original spider queen, debuting decades before Scarlett Johansson stuffed herself into a tight, shiny, black jumpsuit as Marvel's superhero the Black Widow. And I wasn't fictional. I was real.

I never spent one second crafting The Black Widow persona. It was all organic. I did nothing but be myself. I was demure and sweet off the table, but on the table, something swept over me. I was aloof, intense, confident, ruthless, and it all came naturally.

> "First off, Jeanette is stunning, physically stunning, and she dressed the part, and she understood it. As The Black Widow, she stalked the table; I mean stalked the table. When she was competing, the eyebrows would come down. It was dark. It was focused, and she was going to kill her opponent."
>
> —Tom George, Lee's longtime manager

For the first couple of years as The Black Widow gained popularity, I handled media and marketing mostly on my own, with a little help from local billiard clubs.

But when I became the No. 1 pool player in the world, I was overwhelmed by the media circus and frenzy, the nonstop phone calls and requests for appearances. The media loved me, an unlikely national superstar in a sport that wasn't mainstream.

I was a real-life precursor to *The Queen's Gambit*. But instead of a girl who faced adversity at a Kentucky orphanage and went on to become a chess superstar, I was a girl who faced adversity inside a co-op building in New York City and became a pool star.

In the mid-90s, major contracts and deals were coming my way, and I had no idea how to negotiate them. I knew I needed to find top-level, legitimate representation, not some local billiards manager or promotional guy at the pool hall.

I found a sports agency called Advantage International, which was recommended by a friend of mine, an NBA player named Travis Best. Travis told me wonderful things about the agency, now named Octagon, and he told me to call Tom George.

Travis's agent called his boss, Tom George, who promptly said no. There is an axiom in the marketing business that if a client is recruiting you, you don't want that client, because they are desperate. Tom hadn't found me. I had found him.

And by the time I came calling, he had already dabbled in the women's pool circuit, representing Ewa. In the two years Tom represented her, the No. 1 women's player in the world, Ewa landed an instructional billiards book and did a tour for Foster's in Australia. Tom said it was too much work for too little money.

I couldn't take no for an answer, so I flew to Alexandria, Virginia, where Octagon's corporate office was located.

> "I didn't want my staff to waste their time, so I met with Jeanette myself. I could have pawned it off, but I said, 'No, I'll do it. I'll be nice. I'll tell her again in person I'm not interested, and that will be that.' And then she comes into that room looking like Jeanette."
>
> —Tom George, Lee's longtime manager

I walked into the Octagon conference room wearing a nice, form-fitting outfit with a waistcoat. Tom was there with Travis' agent, Andre Colona.

I deny what happened next, though Tom is adamant, and claims he has to verify his version. He says I walked into the room and made a big show of taking off my coat, daintily putting it on the back of my chair, and then sitting down with a flair of drama.

I don't recall any of that. I was just there to do business.

But minutes after I sat down, it wasn't going well. Tom told me it didn't make sense for him to represent me, that there was no money in women's billiards. He told me "no" as nicely as he could and every which way he could.

I kept coming at him. Tom said "no" again, and I gave him a reason he should represent me. Tom said "no" again. I gave him another reason. Tom said "no, no, no, no." But, I wasn't going to be rejected. I was like one of those persistent, annoying salespeople. I was selling Jeanette Lee, The Black Widow, to Tom.

I made him an offer.

"I will bring you the deals," I told Tom. "All Octagon has to do is negotiate them and take care of the legal side of things."

Tom eventually, and reluctantly, agreed. He told me he would represent me, but he would do nothing proactive. He wouldn't be out hunting deals or appearances or sponsorships. That was fine with me. Tom had said yes, and I was on cloud nine. I was giddy and visibly thrilled.

"Relax, relax, relax," Tom said to me. "You had me at waistcoat."

Waistcoat or not, I'm pretty sure Tom never regretted taking me on as a client.

In the early days of our relationship, Tom called me the "human lead machine." Tom said I had an incredible vision of what should come next, and that I was always two years ahead of things. I was bringing him so many potential deals that he didn't have to look for anything. And those leads weren't always just about me.

I would go to every charity billiard event and party I was invited to—paid or unpaid. I went out of my way to find out who the most important people or media contacts were and find a way to come up with ideas for potential business or news pieces. Most of those guys weren't really interested in me commercially. I would have to convince them, at the very least, to get their business card and then hand them off to Tom. I, unknowingly, helped generate all sorts of other opportunities for Tom and for Octagon's other athletes.

Within six months of our initial contract, Tom was hooked on The Black Widow persona. He started handling all of my marketing and media. Tom loved that everything was organic. There was no need to coach me to be anything other than who I was, a fierce, fearless opponent at the table wearing black.

Very soon, The Black Widow blew up.

> "I'd love to take credit for some of this crap. But her showmanship was all natural. All natural. I protected what was there, I exploited what was there, and people fell in love."
>
> —Tom George, Lee's longtime manager

I remember the love. It was intense. I would go to a restaurant with my family and the fans would descend on my table, trying to strike up conversations as I ate a Caesar salad and sipped iced tea.

I would rush to the restroom to get a moment away to breathe, but the fans would follow me. As I hovered inside the stall, they would pass me pieces of toilet paper, asking for autographs. I remember thinking, "What is this? Who am I? Who have I become?"

In my mind, I was just Jeanette Lee, a lonely, outcast girl. But in those moments, that girl felt like a wonderful stranger to me, someone who was truly loved.

Inside the pool halls, the crowds roared and fawned over me. They made me feel like a superstar. No matter who I was playing, the crowd was always on my side. Always. The whole room rose and fell on my shots. When I missed the pocket, there was a hush. When I made the shot, the crowd rejoiced.

I would stay for hours after tournaments, signing autographs and playing pool with the fans. I was no longer Jeanette Lee. I was this brave character named after a ruthless spider who was absolutely idolized.

> "If you're talking to someone and you mention that you're the sister of The Black Widow, that person's face totally changes.

> It's like, 'Wow, oh my.' They are not talking to a human being anymore. They are just talking to a symbol of something."
>
> —Doris Lee, Jeanette's sister

I was a symbol of something. I was a symbol of a powerful woman, a first-generation Korean American who, through my career, racked up more than 30 national and international billiards titles, millions of dollars in earnings, and unheard-of fame for a professional pool player.

I was a symbol of feminism, at least that's how I see it, a woman playing a man's sport, wearing sexy black clothes, and dominating the game. I was The Black Widow.

And the women hated me.

CHAPTER 13

PRETTY DOESN'T MAKE THE BALL FALL IN

THE BLACK WIDOW IMMEDIATELY HAD HATERS. And 99.9 percent of those haters were women.

When I walked into tournaments, every head in the pool hall turned my way. The male fans would swoon, the female fans would stare with admiration, and my opponents would roll their eyes, whisper, and give me fake smiles as they shook my hand.

The women players hated everything about me. They hated the way my long, shiny, black hair flowed down my back. I would swing it around as I descended on the table, ready to take my next shot. They hated my nails, always long, pointed, and perfectly painted.

They hated my glitzy, studded earrings that hung three inches down my neck, and the black glove I always wore on my left hand, decorated with a red spider.

And they especially hated my wardrobe. Of course, my wardrobe was always black, sometimes with an open neck, open back, tight, and in my opinion, never inappropriate.

> "I mean, oh my goodness, how tight can you wear something? How low can you wear something?"
>
> —Loree Jon Jones,
> eight-time world champion who was on the WPBA
> dress code committee, in *Jeanette Lee Vs.*

The women scoffed, too, at the shoes I wore, spiky heels and thigh-high leather boots. "I can't even walk in heels, much less play pool in heels," Loree Jon said.

The women on the tour wore outfits that made them look like librarians, preachers' wives, and schoolteachers. I always believed that you didn't have to look prudish, dress like a man, or play like a man to be a badass at pool. The women seemed to disagree.

"We didn't want to be known as just kind of the sex thing and then it was over tomorrow," Ewa Mataya Laurance, a WPBA Hall of Famer, said in *Jeanette Lee Vs.* "Every appearance I did, I had a business suit on. This is about the sport. We're selling longevity. We were trying to get respect."

If you look at my videos, I don't think I ever dressed in a way that was disrespectful to the sport. We also had a dress code in place that didn't allow it, but my reputation ran ahead of me. But the women players saw me as a threat, as an outsider, as a cocky opponent who was blazing my own path, a selfish path that didn't include them.

I came on the pro tour as a rookie in the early '90s, when the sport of women's billiards was finally getting some recognition and respect. The women were no longer just a sideshow to the men's events. They were holding their own major tournaments and they were on a mission to grow the sport together.

The women players were all for one and one for all. Nobody got favoritism, nobody was the star, and nobody was supposed to stand out from the crowd. It was a well-oiled, conservative, modest machine.

It was a boring machine, in my opinion. And I paid for not following the pack.

After tournaments, I would go to restaurants where the women players drank and talked pool. I would sit alone at a table, listening to their laughter, feeling like an outcast once again.

None of the top women on the tour would even acknowledge I was there. They never looked my way. They never asked me to join them at their table.

Eventually, I would leave the restaurant and go back to an empty hotel room, still hearing their laughter echoing in my head. As I sat in bed staring at the television, I would wonder if the women were back at the restaurant bashing me. I knew they were.

> "Jeanette was not well liked by the women. They were incredibly jealous of her."
>
> —Don Wardell, Lee's longtime physician and friend

The women had an opportunity to welcome me, mentor me, and teach me. They had an opportunity to rally behind me and make me one of their brightest stars. Instead, they tried to push me down and hide me between the couch cushions.

I never understood why the women didn't like me. I never said an unkind word to any of them. I never bashed them in public, and I never taunted them as I demolished them on the table. I wasn't cocky. I didn't think I was better than any of them.

JoAnn Mason was the cocky one. It was very hard to like JoAnn, a pretty, blond, stone-faced woman nicknamed "The Battling Beauty." JoAnn was always polite, but it was in a very holier-than-thou way. Terse, staccato words came from her mouth. "Hello, Jeanette." "Good luck, Jeanette."

JoAnn had been a child prodigy of billiards in the 1970s on the East Coast pool scene, born in the The Bronx, and raised in Monticello, New York.

By the time she was 13 years old, JoAnn was trouncing grown women at the table. She won the WPBA Big Apple Amateur 8-Ball title just before she turned 14. She joined the tour a few years later and, at 21, she clinched her first WPBA title, winning the McDermott Masters in 1988.

By the time I was on the tour as a rookie, I would see JoAnn at regional tournaments and it felt like she, literally, was looking down on me. Until the day I drew her in a tournament and had to play her in a race to nine wins.

As we played our match, I wanted nothing more than to prove to JoAnn that she should not be looking down on me. Instead, I sucked. I played terribly.

JoAnn, who was ranked No. 2 in the world at the time, was so intimidating. She quickly got me down 8–1. Then, something ignited inside of me. I was not going to let JoAnn annihilate me. I was going to prove myself to her.

I scratched and crawled my way back to tie JoAnn 8–8, then lost 9–8. That was one of the few losses I ever had that I was actually proud of. I had come back from what seemed like a sure defeat and showed just how great of a pool player I was. I had shown just how much heart and grit I had.

The pool table was the only place I felt that way. Most of my life, I had no self-esteem. It was ingrained in me that I was not enough, that I was not good the way that I was. That came from those early years when my classmates would taunt me for being Korean and for having scoliosis.

When I looked in the mirror, I didn't like what I saw. I didn't have incredible eyelashes. I didn't have any standout features. I was just barely average.

But as I played pool, all these people, the fans and the media, started calling me beautiful. And my female opponents seemed to latch on to that. They seemed to think of me as nothing more than a pretty face.

As I rose to a top women's player, I made a request to become a board member of the WPBA. I was promptly told no. "We really appreciate that, but it's so important for you to be available for the media. I think you should leave the board stuff to us. You just go out there and be pretty," the women on the board told me.

That really hurt my feelings, that the women didn't seem to understand that I was a really good player who deserved respect.

Pretty, after all, doesn't make the ball fall in.

> "Jeanette was gorgeous, but she had this incredibly competitive side. You've never met anybody this competitive—unless you've met Michael Jordan. It was that level. It was, 'If we're keeping score, I'm going to have to rip your heart out.' She was just fearsome, and that intimidated a lot of the women."
>
> —Don Wardell, Lee's longtime physician and friend

For the most part, the women's hostility toward me wasn't overt. It wasn't like they spewed hateful words or belittled me publicly. Mostly, it was passive aggressive—avoidance, terse greetings, and forced words of congratulations when I trounced them on the table.

But the women didn't have to be overt. I always felt their resentment. And sometimes, they made it known.

When Allison Fisher accepted her trophy after beating me in the Brunswick Delta Classic Championship, she looked back at me holding her trophy up and taunted my smaller trophy, singing out, "Mine's bigger than yours."

Years later, Fisher admitted she was "a little envious" of me. She was the No. 1 player in the world at the time, yet she didn't have the fame I had. Fisher was known as the Duchess of Doom, but it was my persona that captivated the media.

The women hated that. They hated the idea of The Black Widow. And they hated, even more, that I was beating them. I was talented, skilled, an intense competitor, and I was ruthless.

The women players would tell me they didn't think it was right that I used my sexuality as part of my play. They scoffed at what I was wearing. But, 10 years later, those same women were dressing just like me. I never understood why the women thought they had to wear men's business suits to be recognized as strong, beautiful, and skillful at what they did.

> "The first time I saw Jeanette, she was the absolute antithesis of what the women's classic tour branding was supposed to be at the time. I had women actually tell me, 'I don't think she's good for the women's tour. I think she's a step backward.'"
>
> —Mike Panozzo,
> publisher of *Billiards Digest*, in *Jeanette Lee Vs.*

One Christmas, I went to my mailbox and found a package from one of the top women players on the tour. I couldn't believe it. Maybe I was wrong about the way they felt about me. I tore into that padded envelope, only to find the gift was a copy of the Dr. Seuss book *Yertle the Turtle.*

Inside, on the cover page, was a handwritten note from a player I won't name: *I think you will connect with this book. I think you will connect with Yertle.*

In the book, Yertle is a self-absorbed creature, obsessed with being the loftiest turtle in the kingdom. He eventually demands that other turtles stack themselves beneath him, so he can sit atop the highest throne. As he revels in glory, the turtles beneath him, holding him up, are in pain.

That book was about how you step on people, without any compassion, to get what you want. When I got that package, I realized that's what the women thought of me, that I was only out for myself.

"The difference between Jeanette and me," Allison would say, "is Jeanette always wanted to be known as the most well-known player in the world, and I wanted to be known as the best player in the world."

Allison was wrong. It was never about being well-known or famous. Those women misunderstood me. I didn't care about Jeanette Lee getting notoriety. I wanted to be the best in the world just like they did. It had nothing to do with fame.

I just had this deep love, this raging passion to play pool. And to play pool, I needed sponsors. And to get sponsors, I needed to be marketable.

The Black Widow was the answer.

When I came on the scene, 30 years ago, making a living playing pool wasn't possible in the women's game. You had to come in second or third in a tournament to even make a penny after you covered your travel expenses.

Most women had second jobs. My second job was the endless hours I spent working the phones, trying to brand and market The Black Widow.

I soon began pulling in high-dollar sponsorships from the billiards industry and outside of it. I was the first pool player, man or woman, to transcend the sport, landing deals with companies like Bass Pro Shops that had nothing to do with the game. I was making appearances on late-night talk shows, morning news shows, in newspapers, magazines, and in trade publications.

I was a star on ESPN2. It was the women's tour that helped create ESPN2, a fledgling station that needed programming. The WPBA had plenty of programming to offer, and we became something that people wanted to watch.

ESPN2 made sure people were watching me. They literally made me a superstar.

> "Nobody knew who Jeanette Lee was until she went on ESPN. And then, boy, did they know who she was. This wasn't Minnesota Fats walking in."
>
> —Mark Patrick,
> former Indianapolis television sports anchor,
> who covered Lee

As I entered a pool room for those tournaments that aired on ESPN on the weekends, it was a massive production. I would stand with a cue in my hand as my name was announced to a cloud of colorful smoke erupting behind me.

As I walked to the table, men would stretch out their arms to try to get high fives from me. I would saunter to the table, and break a rack of balls with such force, I jumped off the ground to raucous cheers.

I never wanted to be vulgarly sexy, like that over-the-top cartoon character Jessica Rabbit in the movie *Who Framed Roger Rabbit?* I wanted to be alluring like Catwoman. But sometimes, people didn't see it that way. They seemed to think I was Jessica Rabbit.

I was just proud to be a woman, and I had no problem celebrating the things that separated the women from the men. I sometimes watch my old matches from the mid-90s and look at what I was wearing, and I still don't think I was ever dressed inappropriately.

I always wore slim-fitted outfits that hugged my body for a few reasons, including the game. The rule on the pool table was that it was a foul to strike, touch, or make contact with the cue ball or any balls in play with anything other than the cue tip—the body, clothing, chalk, or cue shaft. So, if you were wearing a loose blouse that contacted a ball, it would be a foul, meaning the ball went to your opponent.

I was also a New Yorker in my early twenties. There was no way I was going to play in pleated slacks, which is what most of those women were wearing back then. I liked my dress to be clean, confident, feminine, edgy, and strong.

That was the point of my look. I always thought it was okay for a woman to dress very feminine, to celebrate her own curves, and to be comfortable with her own body. Some people thought it was just to attract men, but not every woman's life revolves around men. Mine sure didn't.

If I was going on tour with a bunch of women, with no men around at all, I still would have dressed the same way, because I dressed in a way that made me feel beautiful and strong, and that's what mattered to me.

And I promise you when I stepped into the arena to battle Allison Fisher, being sexy for men was the last thing on my mind. I was determined, ready, focused, and hungry, all while being a strong and beautiful Asian woman, and people didn't seem to understand that.

At one TV appearance with a woman reporter, she began the interview by saying, "It's Jeanette Lee. Thank you so much for being with us, and the crew thanks you for wearing that outfit."

I was taken aback. What was this about? I was wearing a black jumpsuit, gathered with a belt at my waist, and a top that reached up to my neck, baring my right shoulder.

"You're obviously a very beautiful young woman and you don't hide that fact with the outfits," the reporter went on to say.

I stepped back laughing, and looked down, saying sweetly, "This is a nice outfit. My shoulder. It just shows my shoulder." But before I could get the words out, that reporter talked over me: "Hey, if you've got it, bump it with a trumpet."

It seemed I always had a target on my back. People, especially the women, wanted to find something to bitch about.

> "The WPBA was a very close-knit little family and very together and, when Jeanette came on the scene, it was like a bomb coming through. 'Here I am.' You kind of sat back and said, 'Please. Who is this person?'"
>
> —Loree Jon Jones,
> 8-time WPBA world champion,
> in *Jeanette Lee Vs.*

The women never tried to get to know me. If they had, they would have known I wasn't the person they were reading about in the media. The articles written about me always centered on The Black Widow persona, the woman who wanted to eat her prey alive.

The media would take my words and twist them to fit this character they watched at the table. That was frustrating sometimes, but I'm not sorry they did that. The media helped build The Black Widow from the ground up.

After that article in the *New York Times Magazine* (the one from my first ever pro event that branded me "the bad Bond girl," while also throwing out phrases like, "vampish appearance," "exotic," "see-through black, netted blouse," and "satin bustier"), all hell broke loose—in a good way.

As I said, Ewa Mataya was the focus of that article and the one on the cover of the magazine. After that, she and other women players were suddenly on the radar of mainstream media. It was a spark that ignited a following for the women's tour.

My following grew, too.

> "Jeanette became so popular, and the women hated her, but she was also the player who was making their sport popular.

> She was, in a way, their biggest ally. The women never, ever, gave her any credit for that."
>
> —Tom George, Lee's longtime manager

But no matter how I tried to help the women's tour, it always felt like I didn't fit into the women players' plan. I knew they didn't want me at the tournaments. They felt like enemies to me, and I cried. I cried all the time. I was still a kid, after all.

I was in my early twenties, thrown in the middle of a bunch of adult women who were acting like junior high kids. It was horrible. I have very bad memories from that time, very dark moments.

All I wanted was to be liked. I wanted to be accepted. I looked up to those women and they were judging me without even knowing who I really was. That bothered me so much, and it still bothers me to this day, just how badly I was treated coming onto the tour.

I partially blame the media for that.

During an interview for one newspaper article, I was asked what went through my mind as I hovered over a table, with my signature furrowed brows and intense look. I told the reporter how honored I was to be playing pool at this level, and how I looked up to the women pros.

Then I told him that once I was at the table, something came over me, and it was "either get out of my way or get stepped on."

The article came out, void of the kind words I had said about my opponents, with a headline that read: "Get Out of My Way or Get Stepped On."

That's how the women saw me and, as far as they were concerned, they were justified in their hostility toward me. Their side of the story was always that I was too cocky, but they could never say that I said a cocky word against them.

They just saw all of these articles where I was outspoken about what I wanted to accomplish as a player.

> "The women resented her, especially the ones who were better players and winning more often, because Jeanette was getting all the glory and the jingle. And you couldn't even hate her, effectively, because she was always sweet. If she had been a jerk, then you could hate her, but she never was."
>
> —Tom George, Lee's longtime manager

I never felt like I fit in on the women's tour. I was either hated or respected, but never family, never really a part of the group, and that was hard. There were cliques of women and they would all hang out. I never felt comfortable enough to join them.

Instead, I would befriend the strays, players like me who didn't fit in. I became very close to Helena Thornfeldt, who was known as "The Sledgehammer" because of her massive break. The women on the tour never warmed up to Helena, a Swedish-born player who became a WPBA U.S. Open winner, as well as runner-up at the 1996 Women's World 9-Ball Championship.

Helena was inducted into the WPBA Hall of Fame in 2017 and, in 2019, finished ninth at the WPBA Masters just months before she died by suicide at the age of 52.

When I learned of Helena's death, it hit me hard. I started thinking back on my days with her, how we were two lost souls who loved billiards, how we just wanted to be welcomed by our competitors. And how we never felt welcomed by the other women.

Now, when I go back to the tour, most of those women who were hurtful to me are nice. They are kind. But the way I was treated by them in my early years affected me. I promised myself as the 21-year-old Jeanette Lee that I would make sure no other player ever felt like I did—alone.

Once I became a champion, I always made it a point to go out of my way to meet the rookies. I would say hello, introduce myself to them, talk with them, and mentor them. Many of those players stayed on the tour and became great competitors.

Through the years, some of those women have come up to me and told me I was the first pro to welcome them, to talk to them, and they are grateful for what I did. That feels good. I wanted to be the change I wished to see in the world, to change the way that I was treated.

I know that if the women players had talked to me in person, really talked to me, and gotten to know me, they would have seen that I absolutely did respect them.

They would have learned there are two sides to me. There is the competitive person who works her ass off and plays with confidence. And there is the down-to-earth, very nice, sometimes insecure Jeanette. Never cocky.

There was no way I could be cocky, no reason for me to be arrogant because, unlike the other women on the tour, I was getting my butt handed to me every day by the men of New York City. Even when I became a top-ranked player and I was beating the pro women, I couldn't touch the pro men.

I owe a whole lot of my success to the women players who pushed me and made me want to beat them, to show them that I was not just a pretty face.

But I owe a lot of my success to the men, too. Not just the players who took me under their wings and played against me at Chelsea Billiards and all those other pool halls, but the male fans, the male reporters, the men who said unsavory things to me.

And the men who made me a bona fide sex symbol.

CHAPTER 14

THE MEN: THEY SEXUALIZED ME, MENTORED ME, AND GAVE ME HUMILITY

I WALKED ONTO THE SET OF COMEDY CENTRAL'S lewd and crude *The Man Show* in 2003, wearing tight leather pants and a black tank top as TV cameras recorded every move I made, zooming in on every curve of my body, capturing every enticing view they could get.

I was in my early thirties and, by that time, I was not only a pool icon, but I had become a veritable sex symbol to men.

That was never my intention, to lure the opposite sex, to make them drool as I played billiards. It just happened organically, and I soon realized I had a pretty powerful weapon at my disposal. And so, I used it.

> "If Jeanette Lee were the checkout girl at a grocery store, you'd still go, 'Wow.' But then you put best female billiards player in the world on top of that, and that becomes

> a fascination. I think, with the men, especially, the entire package was just so incredibly appealing."
>
> —Mark Patrick,
> longtime television sports anchor in Indianapolis,
> who covered Lee

When Jimmy Kimmel and Adam Carolla, the two co-hosts of *The Man Show*, asked me to be a featured guest for an episode, I agreed. As I walked up to the pool table, under the glitzy, glaring lights of the TV studio for my introduction as the show began, I banged four balls in with one shot.

"Very cute with the tricks here," Kimmel said. "But how do you do when it comes to a real game, little lady, against a couple of men?"

Little lady? I had picked up a cue as a teenager, gone pro at 21, and was ranked No. 1 in the world by the time I was 23. I was a billiards veteran. I knew this little lady would not have an ounce of trouble taking out Kimmel and Carolla. I leaned over the table to take my first shot.

"So, when I'm watching you on the ESPN shows, there, right there, where you bent over," Kimmel said, "there's the point where I start masturbating."

That comment made me cringe, but I smiled sweetly. I was here for publicity and any "positive" publicity was worth doing.

> "I have almost no interest whatsoever in women's sports unless, and this is a big unless, the women playing the sports are hot."
>
> —Jimmy Kimmel,
> *The Man Show*, featuring The Black Widow,
> March 2003

I quickly learned what I had already suspected. My looks and my body were clearly going to be the focus of this show. Of course,

I wanted to be good for the sport. Even though their "on-camera" crude comments made me cringe, as far as I could tell, they made themselves look crude and ignorant. They knew it and I knew it. As long as I behaved with class, they couldn't hurt me. It was an entirely new audience that now knew about professional pool, and The Black Widow. Bringing new eyes to the sport, in any way, was good for the sport. And the men? They helped me every step of the way.

If not for the men, the men who were always welcoming, sometimes degrading, sometimes loving, sometimes disgusting, sometimes the most wonderful people on Earth, I would not be where I am today.

Pool was a man's sport when I started out in 1989, and it's still a man's sport 35 years later. Just look up any official billiards stat on gender and the game, and women are, overwhelmingly, in the minority. Men have been, and still are, the major force on the green felt table.

I have always hoped that my three decades on the pool scene played a little part in making the game a woman's sport, too. A 1997 study conducted by the Billiard and Bowling Institute of America found that the number of female pool players had grown at a rate of 25 percent since 1987, while the number of male players had grown at a rate of 17 percent. In 2002, the BBIA honored me with the prestigious BBIA Industry Service Award. I was only the fifth woman to receive this award since its inception in 1954.

If I played even a small part in bringing more women into the game, I have a lot of men to thank for that—good and bad.

There were the men at the pool halls who embraced me as I worked on my newfound passion. They played pool with me and gambled against me. There were men who managed the pool-table rentals that chose to comp my table-time bill. There were men who sponsored my tournament entry fees. There were the men who looked out for me when I left a dark billiards club at night. There were the men who shooed away the gross, gawking predators.

And there were the men who told me I was worth something, that I really was good, that they were proud of me. And for some reason, when those men told me that, I actually believed them. I believed I was worth something.

But there were also the men who sexualized me. There were the men who exploited me. I know that was wrong, but they may have helped me more than anything.

As I rose to fame, I used my skills, along with my sex appeal, and the men ate it up.

> "Jeanette does have a very strong sense of crowd. She gives them what they want. She's just sexy enough to be sexy, but not so sexy that she's off-putting. She would flip her hair and, when she was playing men, she flirted with them, trying to get them to miss."
>
> —Tom George, Lee's longtime manager

On *The Man Show* in 2003, as I trounced Kimmel and Carolla on the table, they took breaks drinking beer, watching me as they pretended to read books on how to pick up hot Asian chicks.

I didn't back away. I kept up with the act. And I showed them just how good I was. "You bitch," they said as I hit a winning shot.

"You told me not to touch your balls," I said, knowing exactly what I was saying. "So, I didn't."

Kimmel and Carolla poured talc powder down their pants, saying they needed to "chalk" their cues, and ate pretzels. They called me "honey" and told me to get them beers. Then, when my skills at the table had done all the talking, they finally acknowledged they could never beat me at pool.

"You know what?" Kimmel said to me. "This is ridiculous. You really want to play some pool? You want to play pool my way?"

"I'll play pool any way," I told him. The show ended with me lounging in a swimming pool, wearing a black bikini, as Kimmel told me the entire gig was a diabolical scheme to get me into fewer clothes. I smiled again.

At the time, there was nothing I could do but smile. I was the spokesperson for the entire sport, especially on the women's side and I felt this responsibility to carry the sport, to advance the sport, and to advance women as athletes. I was a fierce advocate for my gender.

In individual sports, like pool or golf or tennis, it's usually every man or woman for themselves. But at that time, the women of pool were rallying together as one big team, trying to make our version of the sport mainstream. They didn't want it to be some side show and, even if they didn't like it, I was their main act.

> "Rising tides lift all boats. And Jeanette was the rising tide."
> —Tom George, Lee's longtime manager

My fame not only helped advance the women's game, but their value. Every time I made a commercial appearance, made a speech, or showed up for a store opening, I charged a fee. As I became more valuable, raising my fees, the other women hiked up their fees. They weren't making as much as I was, but they were definitely making more than they had before I came onto the scene. I also sometimes took $20 challenge matches with my fans between tournament matches at my booth. Years later, other pros started doing the same thing.

Starring on *The Man Show* was a bit uncomfortable, but the jokes weren't mean spirited. They were just two guys playing sexist idiots, two idiots who wanted the best for me.

Off the set, Kimmel and Carolla were gentlemen, as I knew they would be. By that time, I was no rookie to the male species. I had figured the men out long ago.

By 2003, I had been on the pool circuit for nearly 15 years and, as I played the men to get better, I heard the unsavory comments and chauvinistic jokes. I saw the salacious looks and, maybe a time or two, I felt a man put his hands where he shouldn't have.

I had learned long ago exactly how to determine which men were going to be my allies and which men I should stay away from.

> "Jeanette couldn't go anywhere without a mob of testosterone coming at her. She was stalked everywhere she went. The guys would come up to her, and pool is not a country club sport like golf. The pool fans? I'm not sure pool is even a blue-collar sport. It's a step below blue collar. It's no collar. She put up with a lot."
>
> —Don Wardell, Lee's longtime physician and friend

The men saw something in me, and it captivated them. I was a woman playing a man's sport, and I was good at it.

At the Derby City Classic in 2010, in an arena dominated by men, I won the Louie Roberts Action and Entertainment Award, which no one thought a woman would ever win. And I'm guessing a woman will never win it again.

The Derby City Classic is an annual pool convention and tournament held in January in Indiana, near Louisville, Kentucky. It is eight days long and offers various disciplines of competition for pool players of all caliber. It's my favorite tournament in the U.S. to attend.

The tournament matches were on the main floor of the casino, but upstairs were the "Green Rooms." That's where all the gambling action was. Professionals and road hustlers from all over the world would come to this event. Some would play in the tournaments, some would only gamble upstairs. I was one of the lunatics that would try to do both—while also doing a few public appearances for the casino, playing pool with the fans, and signing autographs. It was exhausting.

But gambling upstairs with the guys, their cash against mine, for as much as $20,000 a set of 9-ball or, at one point, playing $5,000 per game of "one-pocket," another discipline in pool.

The Louie Roberts award is given to the player at that tournament, which features more than 800 players, for their skill and charisma battling it out on the table in the action room. In one match, I gambled all night until ten in the morning, when I was called to play my pro tournament match. I had to stop, hustle my way downstairs, play my match, and then run back upstairs to keep gambling.

One time I started feeling extremely sick. I had gambling matches to be played at a set time, but I was throwing up so much in my hotel room that I couldn't make my way downstairs in time. I sent someone ahead to tell my opponent how sick I was and that I'd need more time. They understood, but all the fans didn't. Some haters complained, calling me a diva, saying I thought I was a big shot as "The Black Widow," and so I could show up for my matches whenever I wanted. What they didn't know—and even I didn't know—was that I was experiencing morning sickness. I was pregnant. Eight months later, at 39 years old, I gave birth for the first time, to Savannah Lee, my beautiful, fifth and last daughter.

I won that award in a landslide, earning more than 90 percent of the votes from my male peers, beating out players like "Strong Arm" John, Harry Platis, and Richie Richeson.

"Jeanette Lee never failed to draw a significant crowd in the action room, an implicit criterion for the award," wrote OnePocket.org in 2010. "Throughout the demanding conditions of the often lengthy battles that took place mostly late at night, or on into the early morning, and frequently with a distracting throng of spectators, Jeanette maintained her grace and elegance while providing a high level of entertainment with her championship-caliber play."

Winning that award was one of my proudest feats, because I showed that a woman could be a contender among the men. The fact that the award was voted on by my peers, mainly men, made it that much more gratifying. I had their respect. I have to say, to this day, there's still nothing better than beating a man in stilettos. There have been plenty of other moments like that, smaller moments, where I proved to the men that pool wasn't just their sport.

In 2000, I played a match against Indianapolis sports television anchor Chris Hagan, who was doing a story on me. He was visibly blown away. Hagan had played a lot of pool in high school and college, and he said he always sized up his opponents based on looks. Until he played me.

> "Jeanette started making shots with her movie star, model good looks. She was cutthroat. She broke a lot of stereotypes. Once you heard her strike the cue ball, you knew this was a real player. This was not an act. She was a world-class billiards player who just happened to be beautiful. This was not a gimmick."
>
> —Chris Hagan,
> longtime sports anchor for FOX59 in Indianapolis

Hagan was one of the good guys. Most of the men thought the women *were* a gimmick, at least in the early years of my pro career. The men were always the main event on the tour, and the women were always a sort of circus side show.

Most of the male pros didn't really consider us pool players. Some just thought it was kind of cute that we were playing. Some hated that we were playing.

There were some men who resented that we were invading their space. At that time in billiards, there were open tournaments, for men and women, and there were women's tournaments, where men weren't allowed. There weren't many men's only tournaments.

"We can't play in their tournaments, so why can they play in ours?" the men would lament. For some reason, just because we had women's events, some guys assumed that any event that wasn't promoted as a women's event was automatically a men's event. When most of the events were open to both men and women, the gender wasn't specified. In fact, if the tournament promoter announced it as a men's tournament, women weren't allowed to play in them either. In any case, for every male player that complained, there were 100 of them that didn't. Most of the men gave us respect, and they welcomed us on the tour.

And there were a lot of men who welcomed me, who mentored me, who were role models to me, and who became my biggest advocates.

One of those men was a guy nicknamed "Flaco." He played at Chelsea Billiards and I really looked up to him. I would sit and watch him play for hours. I always felt comfortable being around him. He never hit on me. He was always a gentleman.

But then, one night, he asked to take me out of the pool hall. I was a little nervous at first. I trusted Flaco, whose nickname in Spanish meant "skinny," but I didn't really know much about him outside of the pool hall. I didn't know where he worked. I didn't know if he was married or had a family. He was just a guy I played pool with.

Flaco told me he wanted to take me to Brooklyn to meet someone special, and I nervously agreed. Flaco was one of the good guys. He wanted to take me to Brooklyn to see one of the best women's pool players around. Flaco just wanted to help me. He wanted me to see a woman who was phenomenal at the table.

Her name was Jean Balukas, and she had gotten her start in billiards at the age of six, as a child prodigy during a pool exhibition in New York City's Grand Central Terminal, where she competed against adults in a way a six-year-old shouldn't compete.

Soon after that appearance, national television shows came calling for Jean, including CBS's primetime program, *I've Got a Secret.* By the age of nine, Jean had placed fifth in the 1969 U.S. Open straight pool championship, and then she nabbed fourth and third place the following two U.S. Opens.

Jean was fearless, beating up on top pros in their prime. She won seven consecutive U.S. Opens from 1972 through 1978, all as a teenager.

All the great male pool players always said that Jean was the first woman to really "play like a man." She had incredible power, aggression, and competitiveness. Jean is widely considered one of the greatest pool players of all time.

I was honored that Flaco wanted me to see Jean. He had watched me at Chelsea Billiards, and he had seen my aspirations to become great. When he took me to Brooklyn to see Jean in the flesh, it felt as if he were saying to me, "You can be this good, too."

I remember being enamored as I watched Jean. I was infatuated. I was going to be her one day. That night with Flaco was a special and pivotal point in my career, the point when I realized that a woman could rise to greatness in billiards, even against the men.

But Flaco wasn't the only man in my life who helped me along the way. There are too many men to name. There was George Mikula, the man I watched that first night I walked into Chelsea Billiards who sent a jolt through me and ignited my passion for the game.

There was Sammy Kong, Tony Robles, Stu the Shoe, Teddy the Greek, Blood, Jonathan Smith, Steve Lipsky, North Carolina Slim, Frankie Hernandez, Ginky Sansouci, Sammy Guzman, Gary the Claw, Nick Varner, Rodney Morris, Bobby Hunter, Mark Wilson, Jerry Briesath, Pat Fleming, and all the other pros that I watched and studied in person or on Accustats videotapes. There were all the men that directed tournaments all around the country that gave me the seasoning I needed to go pro and be fearless against anyone I would face.

There was Greg and Ethan Hunt and the comedian and actor David Brenner, who owned Amsterdam Billiards Club. Greg surprised me by paying for my first official pool lesson by their house pro, Abe Rosen, a great billiards champion who was then in his seventies. Before then, my only pool lessons were by gambling.

There was Mike and Bernie at La Cue Billiards and Cafe, who comped everything for both me and Gene Nagy. They would have custom leather jackets made for me and often kept the room open way past closing so we could get in more time. There was Conleth, who owned Chelsea Billiards and later sold to Telly, who renamed it Slate. Both of them were so supportive. Telly also still owns Bayside Billiards Cafe, which was three minutes from my mom's house. There was Gabe Vigorito of Howard Beach Billiard Club. All of them saw me working hard and chose to support me, gave me discounts, comped my food and drinks, allowed me to practice for free, sponsored me in local and regional tournaments and even some pro events, They also hosted women's billiards tournaments and added thousands of dollars to women's tournaments at my request to encourage more women to compete. These were the guys that drove me to regional tournaments where we would split any money we won. We'd sleep in cars, or sometimes split a hotel room (they'd sleep on the floor). They never, not one of them, ever made an untoward move on me or made me uncomfortable. If anything, they were protective.

There was my friendship with Ira Lee, and later Sang Lee, a world champion 3-cushion billiards player and his partner, professional Michael Kang, who developed my love of 3-cushion billiards. This was where I learned the most about how the cue ball reacts off the balls and the rails. This experience gave me an advantage against the other women, because 3-cushion billiards is not as popular as pocket billiards, so many women didn't understand how to control the cue ball as well as I did.

There was Mike DiMotta, who took a chance on me as a semi-pro when I approached him for sponsorship, giving me a hefty salary and full medical, life, and dental benefits under his group, when no company wanted to give me health insurance because of my extensive medical history. I couldn't have continued on the pro tour if it wasn't for his support.

There was Terry Bell, Larry Hubbart, Greg Fletcher, Jason Bowman, Kevin Hinkebein, Jeff Hayes, and Anthony Spano, all men within the American Poolplayers Association family, who stepped up to help me during my career, but also, especially, during COVID and my bout with stage 4 ovarian cancer.

There was Johnny Morris, whose support allowed me to reach an entirely new audience. He sponsored me, allowed me to participate in Bass Pro commercials, do shows at their Grand Openings, develop my own line of sleepwear at Bass Pro, gave my family tickets to Disney, and flew to see me when I got cancer, donating money to help me with medical bills and to "spoil" myself while I was going through chemo.

There was Efren Reyes, a worldwide pool phenom who was my role model. He played at a different level than any pool star I had ever seen. I always wanted to get to Efren's level, but I never got there, at least not in my mind.

There was Tom George, my longtime manager at Octagon who helped me rise to stardom with his direct, no-nonsense advice. There was George Breedlove, my now ex-husband, who believed in me and fought for me.

There was John Skipper, Magnus Burke, and John Walsh at ESPN who made me a superstar. They paid for my expenses to fly to ESPN and Walsh coached up my announcing skills so that I could possibly do sideline reporting for other sports. They gave me opportunities within and outside of my sport. Skipper helped me further by having Black Widow Marathon Weekends where they would replay my matches back to back on repeat through the entire weekend on ESPN

Classic. They really made me a superstar. They made two *SportsCenter* commercials with me in them—for *pool!* Crazy, huh?

There were the men in three-piece suits who took a chance on me, making me a personality in their companies' advertisements and sponsorships, even if I hailed from a not-so-popular, non-mainstream sport.

There were my two dads, who loved me in the only way they knew how, and taught me a lot—both good and bad. There was my grandfather, a man who gave me unconditional love. There was my first boyfriend, Greg, who put a pool cue in my hand.

There was Cisero Murphy, the first Black professional pool player to ever win world and U.S. national titles. He really stood out to me because there simply weren't many Black or minority pool players competing at a world champion level.

And there was Gene Nagy, the gruff, former billiards champion who turned into a loner, who played me day after day. As he taught me skills at the table, he also helped me ward off the guys.

I had men coming for me, wanting to date me, wanting to take me home. Some of them were great players and, every now and then, one of those guys would catch my eye.

"No, Jeanette. Focus," Gene would say. He was the person who kept me from ever getting involved with any of the guys at the billiards halls. He would tell me it would ruin my career. Even getting back with my ex-boyfriend from time to time, he'd say, "End it, Jeanette. Guys will only be a distraction. Great pool players aren't meant to have soulmates. It's a lonesome journey that you have to take alone if you want to be great. Don't let them slow you down. Trust me. Just focus on pool." He was so very wise.

Soon, I didn't need Gene protecting me from the guys. I had proven myself. The guys at the pool hall stopped saying, "Ooooh, baby, let me show you how to play," and, instead, they started asking to take me on at the table.

Those men, after all, saw me coming in every day, hour after hour, working on my game and playing, and they respected that. They respected *me*.

Instead of hitting on me, they would answer my questions on how to improve my game. Other times, they would just act like they didn't hear me. Taking lessons wasn't as common back then as it is now. Why would they want to help me when they were hoping I'd become their victim? I would ask them for advice. "Why did you do that? How did you do that?" I had only one or two formal pool lessons throughout my entire career, but I did get plenty of tips from the men. Generally, they didn't offer too much good advice. After all, they were starting to see me as one of them, meaning they wanted to gamble, not teach for free. I watched and studied so many great local players. I also had the benefit of so many world champions popping in to play in a tournament, do a trick-shot exhibition, or gamble, like Allen Hopkins, Grady Mathews, Mike Sigel, Steve Mizerak, Jose Parica, Ewa Mataya, Loree Jon Jones, Jimmy Fusco, Danny Barouty, Mike Zuglan, and more. I studied them. I soaked up their games like a sponge. I was so blessed to be able to witness these champions play firsthand—straight pool, 8-ball, 9-ball, 10-ball, one-pocket, and bank pool. No one single person taught me to play as well as I played; I did the work and I asked a lot of questions.

There was Bob Carman, Mark Wilson, and Jerry Briesath, who became my coaches since 1999, developing my stroke to be more consistent and helped me maintain a positive attitude.

And it was those men who helped me become No. 1.

After playing in tournaments and gambling night after night after night against the men, when it came time to play the women, I just wasn't afraid of them. They seemed easy in comparison. Even if I wasn't as good as them yet, I just wasn't afraid of them. There were some women who were beaten before I even shook their hand. I could just tell. I honestly think it was my training playing against all these men. I got so much experience.

> "I was always impressed with how confident and comfortable she was on and off the table. You could tell right away that she was in her element whenever she walked through the door. Jeanette definitely wanted to be there. To see a beautiful, Asian woman like her was very strange for most people, so they didn't know how to react or feel about it. I thought it was awesome because Jeanette brought in an element that had never been seen before. She was beautiful, sexy, super confident, as well as super talented on the table. That intimidated a lot of people."
>
> —Tony Robles, "The Silent Assassin"

The first tournament I ever won, I beat a man in the finals. In fact, every player in the tournament was a man, besides me. It was just some little tournament at some local pool hall, and I don't remember it being an earth-shattering event. But I had beaten the men.

It's strange looking back. I didn't even think about that at the time, that I was beating men playing pool. I never gave myself much credit. In my mind, I was a terrible player with a lot to learn. There were still too many men that were better than me. I was always driven to get better, to be better.

I lived pool, and I breathed pool alongside men. And as I did, I hoped I was empowering other women. Besides boxing, I'm not sure there is a more male-dominated sport than pocket billiards.

Against the high-level men, I didn't have a chance at winning. There was a bigger talent pool for the men, because there were so many more men playing the sport. The male players who rose to the top had to fight harder to get there than the women did.

Amsterdam Billiards Club, aka ABC, regularly gave back to pool by hosting tournaments open to men and women, adding anywhere between $2,000 to $10,000 to the prize fund, in addition to the monies collected from the entry fees of the players. That kind of prize fund drew players from all over the East Coast to compete. They were correct in their strategy to inspire more customers to play pool in their club more regularly by having more opportunities to watch great players. Greg Hunt, one of the owners, was one of my biggest supporters and often would sponsor me in ABC's tournaments, as well as the regional tournaments. I would ask him over and over to put on a women's tournament. He finally said, "I'll tell you what, if you can find 16 women to compete in a tournament here, I'll add $1,000 to the purse."

I was so excited. I was on a mission. I went all over New York City and Long Island to every pool room around. I went to Cafe Society, Chelsea's, the Golden Cue, the Corner Pocket, Bayside Billiards, Deer Park, Jacy's, Soho Billiards, West End, Castle Billiards, and more. There weren't a ton of women playing pool but there were enough. Well over 16, and way more than that of girls and women who would sit in the billiard clubs watching their boyfriends or husbands play. Any time I would see a woman playing pool that could pocket a few balls—and there were plenty—I would introduce myself and tell them that I was recruiting women to play in a $1,000 pool tournament at Amsterdam Billiards Club, on the Upper West Side of Manhattan. I kid you not. I couldn't get eight women to compete. Eight. I traveled to Manhattan, Queens, Brooklyn, Staten Island, and Long Island. It was so disheartening. No one wanted to compete in a women's tournament. They said they weren't good enough and they weren't interested. They weren't that serious. They just liked playing with their boyfriend, etc. It made me sick.

By this time, I'd just started competing on the regional women's tour, called the All About Pool Tour, aka AAPT, based in New England,

and run by Dawn Meurin. She was a touring pro and produced both men's and women's tournaments. We would have anywhere between 20–32 women who drove from everywhere to compete in these events. That was my first taste of competing against just women. I originally doubted I was good enough to compete in a regional tournament where the entry fees were $75. You'd have to have a car to get there and it was a two-day tournament, starting Saturday, and if you kept winning, you'd have to pay for a hotel to continue playing on Sunday. I was only used to playing in local weekly tournaments that I could drive to with entry fees being no more than $20 or $25. For me, it was a big investment and risk, at a time when I rarely had much money. One of my road partners, Sly, convinced me to enter the tournament and offered to drive me, since Dawn often held men's tournaments at the same time.

I finished fourth. And I learned that this was very different than playing in open tournaments, where there were mainly men. Sometimes the top local woman pros, like Dawn, Fran Crimi, Billie Billings, JoAnn Mason, and Nesli O'Hare would compete in the open events with me, but not regularly. But the AAPT were the best women players in the area. I was doing well on the tour so I started making real money playing in tournaments for the first time. Every penny I won was saved to enter more tournaments. A year later, Dawn also started producing Women's Tri-State Tour events in New York, New Jersey, and Pennsylvania. But the events were all outside of the city of Manhattan. I'd learned that I could really compete with the top women. I started winning enough of these events to give me the confidence that I could actually go pro someday.

I wanted more women playing pool so badly. In all of NYC, I'd say I saw 30 women that were good enough to compete with most of the field at the AAPT and Tri-State women's events, compared to the thousands of men that played and the hundreds that competed in the men's events. All the women I'd met by going from room to room when I was trying to convince Greg at ABC to sponsor women's events more regularly, I just couldn't convince them to take the chance. They said they'd be too embarrassed, they weren't good enough. Well, they weren't good enough to compete with the men, but I was speaking to women players that I felt could compete with the local women competitors. They might not win the tournaments, but they were capable of winning matches here and there. They were good enough to compete. I wish I had a good relationship with the other top women in the region, we could work together. But that was out of the question. I felt hated. The women talked about me negatively behind my back and word got back to me over and over. Once again, I didn't fit in.

That didn't stop me from challenging pool legend—and my idol—Efren Reyes to a match in 2001, months after I had won the gold medal in 9-ball at the World Games in Akita, Japan. He's the only man I know that made the other champions' jaws drop. He did things that, sure, maybe the shot was possible, but it was so low percentage that no one would dare shoot it…except Efren "Bata" Reyes. He's known as "Bata" in the Philippines, which means "The Magician."

I traveled to the Philippines to face Efren on his home turf, in a race-to-13 exhibition match at 9-ball. Our battle of the sexes match was advertised worldwide. It was a huge deal, televised, and held live in front of 150,000 fans.

While I was in the Philippines, I was trailed around the clock, not only by fans and 13 bodyguards provided by the government, but by an entourage of reporters. They would follow me back to my hotel room each night, sleep in the hallway, and get up the next morning to follow me out of the hotel.

Efren Reyes may have been known as a "god" in the Philippines, but it kind of felt like I was the "goddess."

Back in the United States, some of the male players resented me for the fanfare that followed me and the notoriety I had.

> "Athletes have this way of being, 'I'm better than you, so I ought to be making more money than you.' There was resentment. You could feel it. You could see it with the guys. She would eat up all the press. She was on the cover of magazines all the time. She blotted out the sun."
>
> —Tom George, Lee's longtime manager

But no matter what I was doing publicity wise, no matter how much more popular I was than the men, they always played better than me. That was just a cold, hard fact. There was no room for me to talk or taunt the women because, every day I was walking into a pool hall and getting beaten by men, some in their twenties and some in their seventies.

I was getting beaten by the men every day. I always knew I had a long way to go, because of the men.

More than anything, I thank the men in my life for believing in me and showing me respect. I thank all the guys that would beat on me at West End or Deer Park or on the Joss Tour.

The men were the ones who kept me grounded, kept me humble, and kept me fighting.

Still, I'm thankful I got the opportunity to compete in the WPBA, even though I always felt hated and misunderstood. They gossiped about me, saying I was conceited, trying to get everyone they could to hate me too. But regardless of what they may have thought, I never felt like I was above anyone. I believed I could beat everyone, and there's a big difference between those two.

Today, I can proudly say that our top women can and often do compete with the men. More and more promoters are inviting both the top men and women to their world events. And the women today are much more welcoming and friendly, and I really hope I was part of that change.

I would often go out of my way to introduce myself to up-and-coming pros. I'd invite them to sit with me for coffee or practice together. I would help anyone who asked, whether practicing with them or giving pointers on everything from pool to marketing themselves. I even helped a few by negotiating deals for them. It took a long time, but I finally felt like I was welcome, because the cruelest women either changed their minds about how awful I was, or they no longer played well enough to keep competing with the rising level of play by the top women. I eventually made more friends. I was more accepted and even respected.

And that gave me courage as I fought another battle, as a minority in the world of billiards. I wasn't just a woman playing a man's sport. I was a Korean woman doing something Korean women weren't supposed to be doing.

CHAPTER 15

DOCILE OR DRAGON LADY? I WAS NEITHER

I ALWAYS STUCK OUT as an Asian American woman playing pool. By stereotypical standards, this was not what I was supposed to be doing, hovering over a green felt table in tight clothing, destroying the competition, putting the men in their place.

I was supposed to be docile and modest. I was supposed to be obedient and submissive. And if not any of that, I was supposed to be one of the other stereotypes of Asian women. A scientist, a math teacher, a doctor—or a dragon lady, domineering and full of deceit.

I was none of the above. I was an Asian American outlier, a fierce, talented, smart, Korean woman making my mark inside billiards clubs all over the world.

> "The first time I saw her, I was flipping channels and my thumb immediately came off the remote control, because I

> saw something that I'd never seen. She was fierce looking, focused, and determined. It was mesmerizing."
>
> —Michael Kim,
> former ESPN anchor, in *Jeanette Lee Vs.*

Asian parents don't dream of their daughter becoming a pool player. My mom certainly never dreamed that. Maybe I'd be an engineer or an orthodontist. Maybe a sweet, loving housewife. Never a billiards queen.

I didn't sit down and pencil all of this out. I never said to myself, "I'm going to become a pool superstar." I don't think anybody does that, especially not a woman, and certainly not the daughter of a Korean mother.

It all just happened organically for me, walking into that Manhattan pool hall, falling in love with the game, becoming obsessed with the game, and becoming a phenomenal player of the game.

I became an Asian American superstar athlete at a time when there were very, very few of us. And I did it at a time when Asians in America were desperately trying to gain respect.

The spring after my rookie season in 1992, the Los Angeles Riots wreaked havoc on America. The uprisings began in South Central L.A. on April 29, after a jury acquitted four L.A. police officers who'd been charged with using excessive force in the arrest and beating of Rodney King.

King was a Black man who was a victim of police brutality on March 3, 1991, when he was beaten by officers during his arrest, following a pursuit for driving while intoxicated on Interstate 210.

If not for a bystander named George Holliday, who filmed the incident from his nearby balcony and sent the footage to a local news station, the world might never have believed King.

The footage recorded by Holliday showed an unarmed King on the ground being brutally beaten after initially evading arrest. Before that, King was shot twice with an electric stun gun, known as a Taser, enduring darts that carried a charge of 50,000 volts.

In Holliday's video, King is shown trying to get up and run, stumbling as an officer takes his baton and hits King on the side of the head. All the officers charged in the incident were White.

The arrest was covered by news media around the world, and it incited public outrage. I was outraged, too.

When the officers were acquitted, the fury intensified, and massive riots ensued. More than 60 people were killed, and more than 2,000 were injured. During the ransacking and looting, more than 2,300 local shops run by Korean business owners were ravaged, and they suffered nearly $400 million in damages, collectively.

The predominant image of how Koreans were depicted during the Rodney King uprisings was of Korean men sitting on rooftops with rifles.

Due to low social status and language barriers, Korean Americans received little aid or protection from police during the riots, and they became central figures in the fight for equality.

The Rodney King verdict, and its aftermath, has been called a turning point for law enforcement and the Black community. But it also has been called the single most significant modern event for Korean Americans.

"Despite the fact that Korean American merchants were victimized, no one in the mainstream cared because of our lack of visibility and political power," Edward Taehan Chang, founding director of the Young Oak Kim Center for Korean American Studies at the University of California, Riverside, told CNN in 2017.

"Korean immigrants, many who arrived in the late 1970s and early 1980s, learned economic success alone will not guarantee their place in America. [The] immigrant Korean identity began to shift. The Korean American identity was born."

And there I was, right in the middle of that transformation, a Korean pool player ready to be America's superstar.

> "Before the riots, I think a lot of Korean Americans were feeling like, 'Okay, we're getting some traction here in America. We're getting some acceptance here.' And then they saw it all vanish. Jeanette was out there by herself. A lot of people really didn't understand just how tough it was, what she had to overcome to get to where she is."
>
> —Michael Kim,
> former ESPN anchor, in *Jeanette Lee Vs.*

It is surreal, looking back now, to think that maybe I was a tiny factor in helping to advance the lives of Asian Americans in the United States, a catalyst to bring racial harmony.

I know I didn't do anything earth-shattering. I wasn't a politician or a community leader. I wasn't crafting anti-discrimination laws or advocating for Korean rights on the streets.

But I knew what discrimination felt like. I had suffered racism as a young girl growing up in New York City. People didn't like the way my eyes were shaped. They chanted racial slurs at me. They called me an Asian slut.

But when I played pool, I never felt discriminated against for being Korean. Even as my ethnicity turned heads everywhere I went, the fans were kind and welcoming. America seemed to rejoice in every victory The Black Widow had at the table.

I was showing the country that a Korean American woman didn't have to be docile or a dominatrix. She could be somewhere in between. And she could be a superstar.

When I was appearing on ESPN2 at the height of my career in the 1990s and 2000s, there weren't many Asian Americans on television, and there were even fewer who were elite athletes—very few.

There was Kristi Yamaguchi, who in 1992 became the first Asian American woman to win an Olympic gold medal in figure skating at the winter games in Albertville, Canada. She also won two World Figure Skating Championships in 1991 and 1992.

There was tennis star Michael Chang, who became the youngest man in history to win a singles major at the 1989 French Open at 17 years old. Throughout his career, Chang won 34 top-level professional singles titles, including seven Masters titles. He was a three-time major runner-up, and he reached a career-best ranking of No. 2 in the world in 1996.

There was competitive figure skater Michelle Kwan, a two-time Olympic medalist, who won a silver in 1998, a bronze in 2002, who was a five-time World champion, and a nine-time U.S. champion.

Beyond her athletic prowess, Kwan had a magnetic appeal that captivated the media. Throughout her career, Kwan was one of America's most popular female athletes, landing major endorsement deals and starring in TV specials. She was The Black Widow on ice.

But more than any other sport in the United States, Major League Baseball had the largest representation of Korean Americans. There were players like Chan-Ho Park, a pitcher who spent most of his career with the L.A. Dodgers, and Shin-Soo Choo, an outfielder with the Cleveland Indians (now Guardians) and the Texas Rangers.

None of those baseball players got the media coverage I did. Outside of serious baseball fans, no one even knew their names. Sometimes, when I would pick up a newspaper or magazine and see my face on the cover, I would have to pinch myself.

Why was I one of the few Asian Americans who got to be in the spotlight?

On television, the only Asian actor I can remember, before the 1990s, was the chef on *Happy Days*. Noriyuki "Pat" Morita was a Japanese American actor and comedian who played the burger-flipping, Fonzie-fighting Arnold on the show.

And, of course, there was always Connie Chung. Before I ever dreamed of playing pool, Chung was a Washington-based correspondent for *CBS Evening News* with Walter Cronkite in the early 1970s, during the Watergate scandal. She went on to become an Asian American trailblazer in the media.

At the height of my career, *All-American Girl* debuted in 1994, a sitcom that starred Margaret Cho. The series, loosely based on Cho's experiences growing up in a Korean American family in San Francisco, lasted just one season.

To put it conservatively, Asian Americans were drastically underrepresented in mainstream media at the time, and they still are.

As I played pool, year after year, gaining a following, becoming famous, I was giving many Americans their first glimpse of what an Asian woman was.

> "There are two sets of stereotypes of Asian American women. There's the submissive, the docile, lotus-blossom stereotype, and then, on the other side, there is the menacing and manipulative, exotic dragon lady, somebody who is sexually alluring, but also may be sexually commanding and dominating. Jeanette was absolutely positioned more on the dragon lady side of the spectrum."
>
> —Jeff Yang, cultural commentator,
> in *Jeanette Lee Vs.*

It's true. I was not submissive or docile, and I've been called "dragon lady" more times than you can imagine. But I never felt like I fit that stereotype. I am not menacing and I am not manipulative. I didn't want to be scary and threatening. I just wanted to be fierce. When I looked strong, I felt strong. This sport is very mental, and so is the art of competition.

What I was actually trying to represent in terms of being an Asian American woman was strength, beauty, intelligence, feminism, confidence, kindness, hard work, and compassion. That was important to me because that's what I truly believed I was meant to be.

I give some credit to The Black Widow nickname. I didn't like it at first, because I cared too much about what people thought of me. But that nickname allowed me to stop trying to fit in. It allowed me to set my own path, and create my own community.

I was very conscious of how I looked, and what I represented. And I realized the harder you work to become what you want, the less you focus on trying to please others, or trying to fit in with them.

And as a role model, that was the message I wanted to send, that a woman can be Asian and feminine, and still be strong, smart, and successful. And I wanted to be an Asian American role model, not just to people in the United States, and not just to women, but to people worldwide.

When ESPN launched *SportsCenter* in Asia in 2002, I became a sensation. Not long after, the network came to the United States to film a documentary on me. That documentary aired twice a day for an entire year on ESPN Korea.

I may not have been the Michael Jordan of Korea, but I was knocking on that door.

As I played tournaments, ESPN Asia would preempt its coverage of baseball games to show me. I felt the adoration from the fans and from the Asian media.

> "She was so beloved there. They literally stalked her everywhere she went. She was an icon."
>
> —Don Wardell,
> Lee's longtime physician and friend

But you have to remember, the greatest player in the world, Efren Reyes (widely regarded as the greatest pool player of all time), was also Asian. Efren was a billiards phenom, a destroyer at the table. He was known by the nickname "The Magician" because he made shots that defied physics.

In the Philippines, Efren was probably as famous, if not more famous, than the president. The people there idolized Efren. So did I.

And as I mentioned, in 2001 I got my chance to go head to head with Efren in a 9-ball exhibition match, a race-to-13, on his home turf. I was sponsored by LG Electronics. I had just filmed a commercial in Hollywood for the company's first flat-screen television.

LG Electronics paid for me to travel to Asia for the match against Efren, which was expected to draw more than 150,000 people to the basketball stadium where it was played.

I remember being a little concerned. I'd never been to the Philippines. I didn't know what to expect. And at that time, extremist Islamic groups were invading the southern islands of the Philippines and just about everything had been shut down.

I desperately wanted to go to that match, but was warned that I shouldn't. My manager, Tom George, was very protective of me. I went anyway.

The Philippines government provided me with 13 bodyguards, who picked me up at the airport. I was in shock. Thirteen bodyguards for me? I'm just a pool player. They all wore black suits and had earpieces in. We drove to the hotel, my van in front with two other vans following behind.

The hotel they put me up in was fancier than any hotel I've ever seen, and I've been to some really nice hotels. They unpacked my luggage, hung up my clothes, and shined my shoes.

Everywhere I went, that entourage of bodyguards followed me. Four men in front of me, four men behind me, and five others lurking around looking out for me. They were in the elevators with me, they were outside my hotel door, they were at restaurants as I ate. To be honest, I thought it was overkill because, once I got there, I felt safe. I didn't feel like I was in danger.

Inside that huge stadium, as I walked out to take on billiards legend Efren Reyes, the fans surrounded us, going crazy, trembling, and literally screaming at the sight of me.

There were barricades, but the people were pushing and shoving past them to try to touch me. They would get a finger on a piece of my clothing and shriek. It was the kind of thing you see on TV with real celebrities. And in my mind, I wasn't a real celebrity.

In a way, I felt kind of uncomfortable. But it was also an insane and incredible experience, because I always wanted people to be inspired by me.

I never regretted traveling to the Philippines to take on Efren. I felt this intense love, this magnetic connection with all these fans, who seemed to hang on to my every shot.

I may have lost to Efren 4–13 in that match. But it wasn't a loss, at least not in my mind. In my opinion, he was the greatest billiards player to ever live, and it was an honor to play against him in his own country. And it was an honor to be a role model.

Filipino women got to see me out there competing against a men's world champion. I felt victory in being Korean, being a Korean woman who empowered others.

> "She became a role model for no-holds-barred Asian American womanhood."
>
> —ESPN, in *Jeanette Lee Vs.*

It still seems so crazy to hear people say that I am a role model for Asian women. In my mind, I have always, deep down, been that skinny, insecure girl who was fighting to find her way.

Growing up Korean was never easy. I have never sugar coated that. But as I finally found my way, my purpose, playing pool, being Korean was wonderful, and it was empowering.

Sometimes, I would pinch myself at what I had accomplished. I would think about how I spent so much of my life as a wannabe, watching what everyone else was wearing, what they were eating, what they were talking about, and what they were listening to.

Now, as I focused on my passion, I was the one to beat. I was the one that people wanted to model themselves after.

Had I given up all those years ago, I would never have experienced this sweet victory. I would have never found out how great I could be, how influential I could be, that I could actually make a real difference in life, using pool as my vehicle.

I showed a side of being Korean American to the world that people found refreshing, and they gravitated toward me. The fans gravitated toward me, showering me with affection. The media and big-name corporations gravitated toward me, requesting interviews, and offering lucrative deals.

I was a Korean American woman who could play pool like a rockstar. And that quickly catapulted me from the billiards table to transcending my sport in a way no pool player had done before me or has since.

CHAPTER 16

TRANSCENDING THE SPORT: FROM POOL STAR TO AMERICAN ICON

THE ONLY BILLIARDS PLAYER in America before my time—or after—who landed a major deal outside of the sport was Steve Mizerak, considered one of the best straight pool players of all time.

In 1978, Mizerak was featured in a Miller Lite beer commercial. I was seven years old. I knew nothing about billiards, I didn't know who Mizerak was, and I definitely didn't care about light beer.

But on televisions inside homes all throughout the United States, more than 40 years ago, Mizerak invaded the screen as he sank trick shots at the pool table, sipping Miller Lite from a stein.

Mizerak looked at the camera and told viewers: "Even though a lot of people don't think pool is strenuous, let me tell you something. You can work up a real good thirst, even when you're just showing off."

It was unheard-of at the time for a pool player to make it into a national television ad for a major household brand. Those spots were reserved for NFL players, NBA players, or some legendary, idolized icon like Muhammad Ali.

Fifteen years would pass before another billiards player would reach the pinnacle that Mizerak reached. And that player just so happened to be me.

> "Jeanette was one of those players who really did transcend the sport and bring in eyeballs from outside traditional pool circles."
>
> —Mike Panozzo, publisher of *Billiards Digest*

But unlike Mizerak, I was the face of many brands. My endorsements, outside of pool, included well-known companies like ESPN, Ford, Canadian Club, Frontgate, Reebok, and Bass Pro Shops.

My corporate alliances meant appearances, sometimes pulling in as much as $15,000 each show, for a wide range of major brands: Toyota, Mastercard, Pepsi, Lucas Oil, Netflix, Bacardi, Hewlett Packard, Dow AgroSciences, Spectrum, Gatorade, Maui Jim, and Nordstrom. The list goes on and on.

As I rose to fame at the pool table, I also rose to fame off the pool table. My popularity catapulted me to a place no other billiards player had gone before. Suddenly, I had not only transcended my sport, but I had become mainstream.

> "She had name recognition unlike any other billiards player and unlike most athletes. Jeanette superseded the fame of the sport by a very, very large margin."
>
> —Don Wardell, Lee's longtime physician and friend

Even as my career was growing, I was focused on making money playing pool. The expenses on the tour were high, and the prize funds weren't high enough. I needed bigger sponsors. I was invited to celebrity billiards benefits to play pool with entertainers and athletes from all over the country. I said yes to every invitation to do interviews, play pool, or just show off some trick shots. I had fun, but I was always focused on the prize. So anytime I was at a celebrity event, radio station, talk show, or corporate party, I always made my way around the entire room. I would research and ask questions regarding who would be there and made sure to introduce myself. I gave out and collected business cards. I'd laugh and have fun, but I also made sure that I planted an idea in their head of how we could do business together. I would walk out of every party with 30–50 business cards or notes in my phone, and I would follow up.

I'd throw out ideas; perhaps I could do a show at their national sales conference to thank their top salespeople or help them organize a billiards benefit for charity or do trick shots at their annual Christmas party? And the opportunities came fast. Soon I was going to be on MTV and HBO's *Real Sports with Bryant Gumbel* and in *People* magazine. Hugo Boss and BCBG sent me free clothes and a VIP 50 percent discount so I could wear their clothes during my ESPN matches.

It was hard work doing all that networking, but I loved being involved with anything to do with pool. I loved spreading my joy of the sport across America. And I figured, the more publicity I got, the more marketable I would be to sponsors. Bigger sponsors meant I could stop working my regular jobs and I could just play pool. If I could just play pool, I could get better faster. Major media outlets, television shows, and corporations came after me. They wanted me, a sexy, pool-playing outlier, who was an unexpected star of a mostly straight-laced sport.

I was featured in *ESPN The Magazine's* "Body Issue," mostly naked, and five months pregnant, wearing a tiny, black-netted veil on top of my head that covered my eyes. The photographer had me leaning over the pool table, in just the right position, to cover up the X-rated parts of me.

My photo was part of the feature titled "Bodies We Want." I never knew why anyone would want my body. That photo showed the scars on my back from all the back surgeries I had been through.

The photograph was captioned "Unbreakable." It went on to say that doctors had diagnosed me with scoliosis at a young age and told me I shouldn't bend at the waist. Those doctors told me to stop playing sports, to pick up board games or cards. But I wanted none of that. I wanted to run, and as I got older, I wanted to run the table.

People seemed to love that fight in me. I was this broken beauty who forged ahead bending at the waist, when I shouldn't have been bending at the waist.

I was named one of *Esquire's* Ten Women We Love, Aloette Cosmetics called me one of the Dozen Most Attractive Athletes of the modern day, and I was voted the third "Sexiest Female Athlete in the World" by an ESPN poll of their viewers.

For that article, the reporter asked me to reveal what I thought my sexiest feature was. I took a long pause, a really long pause. "Oh, boy. That's a really good one," I said. "I guess that should be a basic question that anybody should be able to answer, but what's funny is that I don't see myself as sexy...until someone makes me feel sexy."

My then-husband George Breedlove was in the room with me for the interview, so I called out to him. "Honey, what's my sexiest feature?"

"He says I'm not sexy," I joked with the reporter. "No, he said my hair. I don't know if I agree. I never thought of my hair as sexy. I guess a lot of people do, though. I'm known for that jet-black long hair." And I have to say now, as I battle cancer, I really miss my long black hair.

My modesty always shocked the media. After posing questions about my fame, allure, and my beauty, they would look at me aghast as I told them I didn't really think I was beautiful. I wasn't faking my unassuming posture. That's really who I was.

And so it shocked me when huge names in American media came calling for me time and time again. I appeared on *Live with Regis & Kelly*, *The Best Damn Sports Show Period*, *Entertainment Tonight*, *Extra!!*, *Hard Copy*, HBO's *Real Sports*, *The Late Late Show with Craig Kilborn*, the *Today* show, and *The Late Show with David Letterman.*

Letterman sat in his chair, his mouth kind of hanging open as he introduced me walking onto the set. "She's known as 'The Black Widow,'" Letterman said. "Oh my god, The Black Widow." The crowd cheered and whistled as Letterman smiled.

I was a contestant on Korea's *Dancing with the Stars*, appeared on *American Chopper*, *Arli$$*, and I made a cameo appearance in the Walt Disney movie *The Other Sister.* None of those shows had a billiards storyline. They just put me in because, well, I was The Black Widow.

> "Rare across billiards history is the mainstream star. Minnesota Fats was known widely enough to appear on *The Tonight Show* and *What's My Line?* And decades later, Steve Mizerak sank trick shots in a Miller Lite commercial. But neither could ever hold a cue stick to the global reach that Lee—an Asian American woman in a sports world marketed toward men—achieved."
>
> —*Sports Illustrated*,
> "The Little Blessings of The Black Widow," 2021

I made the holy grail of publicity when I was featured in a *SportsCenter* advertisement which, at the time, 20 years ago, was huge.

"It really shows how great you are when you've made a 'This is *SportsCenter*' commercial," Michael Kim, former ESPN anchor, said in *Jeanette Lee Vs.* "I was excited for her because this is a sign that you've made it."

ESPN played a major role in helping me transcend my sport. ESPN agreed to give the WPBA precious programming hours, which gave me the platform to compete and be seen by millions on national television. Specifically, there were several ESPN executives who took a liking to me. Burke Magnus was in charge of billiard programming back then and he found so many ways to use me outside of just watching me compete. When I didn't make it to the final rounds, I was often hired as their play-by-play analyst or I would conduct interviews from the arena. There was John Skipper and John Walsh, who I met at their company Christmas party. The network hadn't planned on having a party that year, but when the sales department unexpectedly exceeded its numbers, ESPN called Tom George. They wanted me at their holiday bash.

Skipper, former president of ESPN, and Walsh, who was known for growing ESPN franchises like *SportsCenter*, ESPN2, ESPN Radio, and *ESPN The Magazine*, took a liking to me.

> "Jeanette's skill and charisma were apparent, and we went all-in on her as an athlete and an icon. It was only natural that we asked her to do a *SportsCenter* commercial. There was not a whisper of protest."
>
> —John Skipper, longtime ESPN president

At my first outing with ESPN, I went to their party and I did my thing, the same thing I always did at my outings. I would give a little inspirational talk, I would do a few trick shots, then for the rest of the three hours or so, I would take challenge matches. People always wanted to say they had played pool with The Black Widow. The women loved that I was such a strong force and so confident. They loved watching me beat all the guys. And the men, well, they all just liked to be able to say they got their balls broken by The Black Widow. If there were kids, they'd look at me like I was some kind of superhero. I don't think I can take much credit for it, but for some reason, I just fit in that little space that worked for everyone.

At my outings, I would demonstrate easy trick shots, and then I would set them up for other people to do. At all my appearances, I always called for the most important person in the room to join me at the table, maybe the CEO of the company or a high-ranking personality.

I would lie the person down on their back on the pool table and put a single piece of chalk in their mouth with an 8-ball on top. I would put a stack of three or four cue chalks as a tower on the pool-table rail with a cue ball on top.

I would then hit the cue ball, make it hit the ball off the person's mouth, and roll into the pocket. The crowd would go wild.

The crowd went wild, too, when I put NFL quarterback Trent Dilfer in his place at an outing I did for the National Football League Players Association. Dilfer who, through his 13-year-career in the league, spent most of his time with the Tampa Bay Buccaneers and Seattle Seahawks, was at that outing, and he was crowing loud enough for everybody around to hear him.

"I'm going to wipe the felt with The Black Widow," he taunted. "There's no way she can beat me. I've got her. You watch."

When it was Dilfer's turn to take me on, the challenger went first. When he broke the rack, not one ball went in. I stepped up and I ran the table on him very quickly. That didn't stop Dilfer.

He got back in line to wait for another chance at me, and he kept boasting. "That's okay. I'll get her next time. She can't beat me twice."

Until I did beat him twice. In our second match, Dilfer made one ball on the break, then missed the next shot. I ran the table again.

> "Sit down, Trent. Everybody was cheering Jeanette on. They got to see something cool, because they got to see her run the balls when it mattered. It mattered because she was putting that guy, that NFL quarterback, in his place. It was awesome. Everybody in that room absolutely loved it."
>
> —Tom George, Lee's longtime manager

Throughout my career, I've done nearly 1,000 outings. Besides corporate appearances, I did a whole series for the military, dozens of them. I went to Guantanamo Bay, all over Asia, all over Europe, all over America, and I played pool with the troops.

Everywhere I went, the soldiers were always respectful, but they couldn't wait to get a chance to play with me. I always let them break first. "This way you're guaranteed at least one shot at the table," I would say to them.

It was all in good fun. I would taunt those opponents who wanted to beat The Black Widow in front of all their bunkmates. Sometimes, I paid the price when I would give one of those soldiers the opportunity to run the last few balls. The place would explode, cheering on one of their own who had taken down a billiards champion who played pool for a living.

Some of the best memories of my life were with those men and women, who were sacrificing their lives for our country. They would tell me how special it made them feel, that I was sent to their bases just to make them feel appreciated. That was a big honor for me.

When I went to Iceland, I arrived at a very small base, maybe 60 people, and a soldier came up to me. "This is such a small base. It's easy to feel unimportant, but just when you think no one cares, no one sees us, we find out you're coming to our base, our little base," he said to me. "Wow, I never thought I'd ever get to meet my idol by serving my country."

Talk about humbling. Just to be part of that was easily one of the most rewarding appearances I've done in my career.

Did anyone ever beat me? Sure, a few got lucky. After all, it's just one rack. That's like someone beating Michael Jordan in a free-throw competition. But, to be honest, those soldiers were the ones that were really impressive because they had access to pool tables at every base. They'd watch pro matches and instructional videos on YouTube and they practiced *a lot*. It made me so happy to see how much they loved the game and how much they appreciated me going overseas to support them.

The guys at the ESPN Christmas party couldn't beat me. But the guys at ESPN loved me.

Soon after that party, the network was asking me to do all kinds of stuff. I would do four or five outings at the Super Bowl, two or three for ESPN, another for Pepsi, another for Gatorade. Each year, the companies changed, but ESPN was always my mainstay, as I worked in the network's hospitality area.

But ESPN and I didn't end with pool. The network had me reporting from the sidelines at ESPN bowling events, Friday Night Fights for boxing, and working their red carpets at events that had nothing to do with billiards, like the *ESPYs*. People started recognizing me, and other marketing offers poured in.

In 2000, my biggest sponsor, Imperial International, connected me with Stern Pinball, one of the world's biggest pinball machine companies. Stern created a game called Sharkey's Shootout that featured my image in glass at the head of the machine, leaning over a pool table. The game was marketed as the first tournament pinball ever, taking place in a pool hall called Sharkey's on Main Street, U.S.A.

"Once a year, Sharkey, the owner, and one of the players, throws out a challenge to all the local talent, and some colorful characters show up to take home bragging rights, and some sweaty stacks of cash," Stern wrote in its marketing of the game. "The current reigning champion at Sharkey's is Jeanette Lee. However, you will first have to defeat five other players at 8- or 9-ball before you have the chance to go toe to toe with The Black Widow."

I still have one of those Sharkey's Shootout pinball machines in my Tampa home. And, stashed away somewhere, I probably still have a few articles of clothing from rapper Jay-Z.

In 2008, I was featured in an ad campaign for Rocawear, an urban lifestyle brand founded by Jay-Z. Inside the pages of the March *Vibe* magazine issue, I was decked out in a sleeveless, hooded, black jacket with white-and-green graffiti splashed on the front.

I remember thinking, at the time, that it seemed my marketability had no bounds. It was unreal to me, and it was amazing to me that I could be at an event with Donald Trump or Muhammad Ali one day, and the next day be at a NASCAR party or headlining an event with an NFL player. And the next day be on a pinball machine or wearing a famous rapper's clothing.

In between my endorsements, licensing, and appearance contracts, I had an instructional DVD called *Black Widow Billiards with Jeanette Lee*, and I landed a deal with a cell phone company, allowing people to buy a photo of me for their phone.

Soon, the money started pouring in. In 2007, I earned about $650,000. In 2008, I earned more than $800,000. There were years, I reached nearly $1 million in earnings, not from playing pool, but from all the extra stuff outside of the sport.

> "Jeanette was no longer a billiards star. She was a sports star. The next level is star, period. I don't think she really ever got to that next level, which only a few people get to. Michael Jordan gets there. Muhammad Ali gets there. Tom Brady got there. I'm not going to say Jeanette got there. She didn't. But she got in the same conversation with all the football, baseball, basketball, and hockey players of her generation."
>
> —Tom George, Lee's longtime manager

Of course, I have to give credit to Tom, and to my agency Octagon, which was a trailblazer in the industry of sports marketing. Originally named Advantage International and later becoming Octagon, it was the first of the big-name agencies to have a unit focused solely on marketing athletes, and that started in 1991, long before any other company joined in.

The strategy at Octagon was to sign athletes across a wide breadth of the sporting landscape, not just big-name athletes in major sports. They looked at less popular sports like pool, tennis, and swimming. Most of the athletes in those sports weren't worth representing, but to cherry pick the top of the top of that niche sport? That had value.

Octagon represented Michael Phelps in 2004, when he won six gold medals in Athens, almost tying Mark Spitz's record of seven golds in one Olympic games.

One year, Octagon had Anna Kournikova, who with Martina Hingis as her partner, won Grand Slam titles in Australia in 1999 and 2002, the WTA Championships in 1999 and 2000, and who became the No. 1 doubles player in the world. Despite never winning a singles title, Kournikova reached No. 8 in the world in 2000.

As doubles players, Kournikova and Hingis referred to themselves as the "Spice Girls of Tennis." Kournikova's appearance and celebrity status made her one of the best-known tennis stars worldwide. At the peak of her fame, fans looking for images of Kournikova made her name one of the most common searches on Google.

Octagon definitely knew what it was doing.

I had no idea how fortunate I was when I signed with the agency in the mid-90s. But I absolutely landed in the right place. If I had signed with a billiards agency or a one-off basketball agency, I never would have gotten the publicity that came my way.

Because of all the different athletes Octagon represented, a wide range of requests came into their agency, looking for an athlete to do X, Y, or Z. Sometimes I fit X, Y, or Z.

Some of them were speaking engagements, some were TV ads, some were corporate appearances, and some were sponsorships. I never missed a single appearance I was supposed to make.

The other agents inside Octagon started recommending me for gigs. I got a reputation inside the halls of the agency that I was an athlete who, if the money was right and the terms were right, I always said yes.

Octagon gave me the nickname, Jeanette "Never Lets You Down" Lee, because if I made a promise to do something or be somewhere, I was going to make sure that happened, come hell or high water—or ice storms.

In January 2000, I had committed to an appearance in Atlanta for the launch of MVP.com, an online retailer of athletic wear and equipment, founded by John Elway, Michael Jordan, and Wayne Gretzky.

But that week, the same week of the Super Bowl in Atlanta between the Rams and Titans, a vicious ice storm struck, and another was set to descend just days before the Super Bowl.

Octagon was canceling all sorts of appearances by its athletes because the talent couldn't get flights to the game. My flight out of Indianapolis for my MVP.com appearance was canceled, too, so I called Tom.

"Oh, don't worry about it. We're getting lots of calls," Tom told me. "I'll tell them. They'll understand."

> "And Jeanette goes, 'No, no, no, no, no, no, no. I'll be there. George and I are already driving. We're halfway across Kentucky now, heading to Atlanta. We'll make it in time.' And I remember looking at the phone like, 'Okay, I'll tell them. They'll be thrilled.' I couldn't believe it."
>
> —Tom George, Lee's longtime manager

My then-husband George Breedlove and I drove 533, very slow, wintery miles from Indianapolis to Atlanta to beat the ice storms. I still remember that eight-hour drive. It was dark and very icy. But I was not going to let them down.

It never crossed my mind to not do everything in my power to be there. I had a responsibility to be there. I had promised to be there.

When I got to that launch party for MVP.com, a crowd gathered around the pool table as a guy walked up to me, introducing himself as Wayne, and said, "Hey, can we play?"

Wayne shot his cue with a cigar hanging out of his mouth. And as we played, news reporters and cameras descended on our table. I was absolutely thrilled. Here I was in a room with Michael Jordan and John Elway and Wayne Gretzky and the cameras were focused on me. I was not expecting to be the person who drew a crowd that night.

After I played Wayne and we took pictures, George turned to me and said, "So how was that? Are you excited that you got to play with him?"

"Play with who?" I asked.

At that moment, it hit George, and he said, "Please tell me you know who he is."

That Wayne I had just battled on the table was hockey god Wayne Gretzky, and I had no idea.

I was so grateful I had made that treacherous wintry drive for that appearance and got to play Gretzky. I always had this incredible passion to do what I said I would do, to be where I said I would be, and to play the match I said I would play, no matter what. Even if I was deathly ill.

When Yue-Sai Kan (the Chinese American television host, producer, author, entrepreneur, and humanitarian, nicknamed "The Oprah of China") came calling, I was ecstatic.

She was the most famous woman in China and she wanted to interview me for her show. After that interview, Yue-Sai became enamored with me in a big way. She decided to do a special billiards event in China featuring three professional Chinese women players and me.

Yue-Sai set up the match to be aired on regional Chinese television, the southern region, which had Shang-Hai in its viewership. It wasn't national, but it was huge. The match was sponsored by a major jewelry company, and it was a big deal.

Yue-Sai had nothing to do with billiards, yet she wanted to hold a billiards tournament. She saw it as a way to empower women, and she wanted me there. I was a powerful woman and I was the biggest star in billiards at the time.

But when I arrived for that tournament, I became very ill. I don't know if it was food poisoning, a virus, or the travel, but I was throwing up. I was dehydrated, and I was more tired than I had ever been in my life.

When I was taken to the hospital, both Yue-Sai and Tom assumed the event would have to be canceled, or at least postponed, and rescheduled.

There was no way I was going to let that happen. I had said I would be there, and so I would be there. I made it from the hospital back to the green room as the first two women were playing their match.

I laid down on a bed with IVs pumping liquids through my body. When it was time for me to play, I got dressed, gussied myself up, went out to the table, and I gave the fans my full Jeanette Lee performance.

After I won the match, I went back to the green room, laid back down on the bed, and got hooked back up to the IVs. I waited, and then I went back out and did the whole thing again. I gave the fans what they wanted. I gave them The Black Widow in full force, and I won the tournament.

I wasn't about to disappoint all those people and, especially, not Yue-Sai, who had put her neck on the line with the TV network. She had planned this whole thing, and the whole thing centered around me. I couldn't let her down.

I always had a sense of obligation to do my job when people took a chance on me, to hire me, to book me for their events, because I knew that booking billiards celebrities was not something that happened every day. I always wanted to under-promise and over-deliver.

Some people have said my fame came because I was beautiful, which of course, I scoff at. I still, to this day, no matter how many times I have been told I am beautiful, do not think I am.

I believe my fame came, in part, because I was always willing to be out there among the people making appearances, doing the 5:00 AM radio interviews or the 7:00 AM morning shows in these little-bitty towns, the things no one else wanted to do. I always said yes and, after a while, it added up to people knowing me everywhere. I was always loyal to every single date I had on my calendar.

And I also believe my fame came because I was actually really good at playing pool.

> "You can be pretty all you want. A lot of people have been pretty and tried to make it. But pretty only gets you so far. You have to win. And winning is what took Jeanette from a pool player getting pool gigs to a pool player who transcended the sport."
>
> —Tom George, Lee's longtime manager

And there is no better example of how I transcended my sport than the deal I got with Bass Pro Shops, a deal which had absolutely nothing to do with pool.

And, yet, it made perfect sense.

CHAPTER 17

BASS, BEAUTY, AND BILLIARDS

I HAD ABSOLUTELY NO CONNECTION or devotion to fishing, hunting, or camping. I was a second-generation Korean American, born and raised in New York City, a very urban existence. My idea of the outdoors growing up was a tiny, green patch of land, or maybe a tract of gravel with a seesaw, in between high-rise apartment buildings.

I never slept on the hard ground in a tent as crickets chirped, snakes slithered, and God knows what other creatures lurked about. I never woke up in the wee hours of the morning and trudged to a lake with a fishing pole, or went to a forest to hunt deer. I never cooked fresh trout in an iron skillet over an open flame. I never went duck hunting. I was not an outdoorsy kind of girl.

I was a woman battling at the pool table day and night in Manhattan, and billiards was an indoor sport. It was played in air conditioning where mosquitoes didn't bite, bees didn't swarm, and where, if I needed a break, I could grab a soda and sit down in a plush chair.

The sport of pool had nothing to do with tree stands, bait casters, bass boats, wading boots, or tents. My sport wasn't an outdoors kind of sport, and I certainly wasn't a flannel-and-denim-jeans-wearing country woman.

But there was a man who came into my life named Johnny Morris, and he was brilliant. And soon my indoor world of billiards collided with the outdoors. Johnny owned Bass Pro Shops, and he found a way to make bass and billiards blend into one big fan base.

I met Johnny at a trade show in the 1990s, where I was working at my modest, no-frills billiards booth. Johnny had his own booth, an explosive display with camping trailers, a fire pit, fishing gear, and race cars.

One afternoon at that trade show, Johnny left his booth and walked to mine. He held his hand out and introduced himself. "I am a big fan of yours," he said. Johnny had been watching me on ESPN2.

> "Jeanette would chalk up and let the hair fall onto the pool table, and, oh my. She was not only beautiful, but she was unbelievably talented, and she had this appeal, this universal appeal. Whether you liked to fish, play the stock market, or play pool, there was something alluring about Jeanette."
>
> —Johnny Morris,
> founder and CEO of Bass Pro Shops

Johnny had once been a bit of an aspiring pool player himself, as a college student attending Drury College. Instead of focusing on his schoolwork, Johnny spent most of his time fishing and playing pool. There was a billiards hall called Campus Cue near the university, and Johnny went there one night, picked up a cue, and he fell in love with the game.

But billiards quickly fell to the wayside as nothing more than a hobby when, in 1972 at the age of 24, Johnny started selling bait and tackle in an eight-square-foot space at the back of his father's liquor store.

As Johnny used his self-taught business acumen and his marketing genius to grow the company, that tiny venture soon became known as Bass Pro Shops, a fishing and hunting retail mecca.

In 2017, Bass Pro Shops acquired Cabela's. Johnny's company also operates White River Marine Group, offering an unsurpassed collection of industry-leading boat brands, and Big Cedar Lodge, America's premier wilderness resort.

Together, Johnny's companies are consistently recognized at the top of major retail rankings. In 2019, *Forbes* magazine named Bass Pro Shops one of America's Most Reputable Companies, based on the public's trust in the organization.

In 2018, the National Retail Federation named Bass Pro Shops the No. 2 Hottest Retailer in America. In 2023, Bass Pro Shops captured the No. 1 spot, and Cabela's the No. 2 spot, as America's Best Retailers in *Newsweek*, with a nod as the retail leader in the camping and outdoor gear industry.

More than 50 years after Johnny started selling fishing supplies in the back of his father's liquor store, today his net worth is an estimated $8.5 billion. "Johnny Morris has earned a reputation as the 'Walt Disney of the Outdoors,'" Bass Pro Shops boasts on its website.

Walt Disney? Yes, Johnny was kind of like Walt Disney to me. He certainly made my dreams come true.

Not long after I met Johnny at that trade show, he invited me as the feature attraction at his booth in Las Vegas for the International Council of Shopping Centers Convention, where developers, landlords, and retailers came together to make big deals.

A pool table was set up as part of the Bass Pro Shops' booth. The developers, leasing agents, and CEOs of big shopping centers would stand in line, waiting for their turn to challenge The Black Widow. Johnny liked that I drew a crowd.

Johnny saw firsthand that I had already transcended my sport, and he saw how perfectly I would fit in with the demographics of his customers. The guys coming into his stores, after all, were the same guys who were watching me on ESPN2.

> "They would go bass fishing in the morning, and go to the pool hall or bowling alley at night. That was the tie. Johnny understood the fact that Jeanette was a good-looking female and she's selling to men 20 to 50 years old. If not for that demographic match, it wouldn't have worked. That's why Jeanette made sense for Bass Pro Shops."
>
> —Tom George, Lee's longtime manager

Soon, Johnny started bringing me to his store openings. Then he put me in national television ads. In the '90s, I invaded homes across America doing TV commercials for the company as a billiards-playing character who didn't know much about the outdoors.

In one commercial, I sat in a camping chair with a tent in the background, next to race car driver and outdoors expert Wally Dallenbach. I had on an elegant, sleeveless, all-black outfit. Wally was in jeans and a red cap.

"Jeanette, can you tell us a little bit about The Black Widow?" Dallenbach asked me.

"Sure, I've won about every major title there is to be won," I said, as my name and the words "Billiards Champion" flashed on the screen. "But really, what it comes down to, is controlling your mind and the stroke."

"Um, that's great," Dallenbach said to me, "but I meant the [black widow] spider."

In another commercial, I stood next to a tree with Dallenbach. "Jeanette, can you spot the poison ivy?" he asked me.

I pulled a leaf off the tree, and I asked Dallenbach, "Is this it?" That leaf was poison ivy.

"You shouldn't touch that," he told me, holding out a can of wet wipes. I quickly grabbed a wipe, and I started scrubbing my hands.

I wasn't acting in those commercials. I really didn't know anything about the outdoors. And I was always up for any publicity. I was always up for anything that got my name out to fans, and out to people who didn't even know they wanted to be fans.

Johnny definitely helped me do that.

> "Jeanette was magical on the table, and she's not hard to look at, either. I felt like maybe quite a few of our customers would enjoy seeing her and being around her."
>
> —Johnny Morris,
> founder and CEO of Bass Pro Shops

For the next four years, I became part of Johnny's brand as a national, integrated spokesperson for Bass Pro Shops. The Black Widow clothing was sold in stores, and life-sized cardboard cutouts of mine welcomed customers through the doors.

I was invited to Bass Pro Shops store openings all over the United States, which featured high-profile celebrities like NASCAR drivers, country music entertainers, Miss Americas, fishing and hunting personalities—and me.

Johnny wanted to draw a massive crowd for those grand openings, not only for his company, but for charity. At every Bass Pro Shops opening, Johnny held an Evening for Conservation. He would donate 10 percent or more of the proceeds from purchases that night to groups whose missions were to save endangered species, protect the environment, conserve and restore habitats, and enhance ecosystem services.

After the ribbon-cutting ceremony was over, different booths were set up to educate people on everything outdoors, as well as booths featuring autograph tables for the personalities Johnny had brought in.

> "Seeing the line of fans that came to see Jeanette, just her pull, really astounded all of us. We had celebrity fishermen like Bill Dance, Roland Martin, and Jimmy Houston, and race car drivers like Dale Earnhardt Jr. and Tony Stewart. But from the very get-go, Jeanette would always have the longest line of folks wanting to get a picture with her. I wasn't the only one watching her play pool on TV, and a lot of our customers became huge fans."
>
> —Johnny Morris,
> founder and CEO of Bass Pro Shops

After the autographs were signed and photos were snapped, people would turn to the pool table. Johnny always had a billiards table at those grand openings. I would put on a microphone and challenge people to a game.

I would tease around with the guys, play easy on the kids, and bond with the women. Johnny said he was always fascinated by how well I engaged with the fans, even as I trounced them at the table.

> "They'd get their balls busted by her, and they still loved her."
>
> —Mike "Karl" Dunham,
> real estate advisor to Johnny Morris

At one store opening that Johnny never wants to forget, and I kind of do, he challenged me to a match. We were in Independence, Missouri, and Johnny, as he always did every time I was around him, and no matter how many times I had beaten him, wanted to play me.

We were battling head-to-head when, before I knew it, each of us had only the 8-ball left. That's when Johnny became really confident, called a double bank shot in the corner pocket…and made it.

The place went wild.

Johnny had beaten The Black Widow. Even with all those championships and tournaments I had won, I couldn't beat Johnny at his Independence, Missouri, store. Johnny said he has always wondered if I let him win that round of pool. I did absolutely nothing to help Johnny make that double bank shot. He made an incredible shot to win.

I never dumped a game to anyone. I'm not that nice. I'm not that merciful. Even if Johnny was the man who was giving me, and getting me, national publicity.

Johnny's marketing plan for The Black Widow worked like magic. Because of me, customers at Bass Pro Shops started falling in love with pool, and pool aficionados soon started falling in love with Bass Pro Shops. Johnny was brilliant. It was his belief that you could cross-pollinate sports.

He would put big dollars into sponsoring race cars, much to the chagrin of naysayers who wanted him to use that money to sponsor another big fishing tournament. Johnny always said his philosophy was simple.

There were a lot of people watching NASCAR races, and if they saw Bass Pro Shops sponsoring a car, then suddenly, to those racing fans, fishing was a cool thing. They would become curious and they would walk into Bass Pro Shops to see what this outdoors retailer was all about.

For Johnny, racing was a way to get his brand out to a larger demographic, engaging with more people. For Johnny, pool was a way to do that, too. And I loved getting to be the person who introduced a whole new audience to the sport I loved.

> "For some people, Jeanette Lee was their first introduction to pool. But as Jeanette played pool, she showed people something else. She showed them her story. She's a hero to me. Some of the challenges she's had in her life, and the adversity? To overcome that is really, to me, extraordinary. She is a champion, not just the inspiration she gave to me, but she inspired so many people."
>
> —Johnny Morris,
> founder and CEO of Bass Pro Shops

In 2009, Johnny and I were at a boat dealers' convention in Branson, Missouri, and all the attendees were down in the dumps. The economy had taken a dive, boat sales were down, and most of the people affected were small, family-owned businesses.

Johnny had invited me to that convention to play pool with the dealers during happy hour, the night before their big formal business meeting. After happy hour, I went out to dinner with Johnny and his wife, Jeanie.

I really connected with Johnny and his wife as I talked about my struggles with scoliosis, about all the surgeries I had endured, and about all the pain I had suffered. The next evening, during the annual gala's dinner, Johnny turned to me and, out of the blue, he asked me to give a speech right then.

Johnny talked about how all these boat dealers thought they had it rough. He told me to tell them my story of perseverance, to talk to them about how, in the big scheme of life, selling a lot or just a few boats doesn't really matter.

> "Jeanette said, 'Johnny I got this.' And she goes up to the podium without a single note, and she tells them her story, from being a young girl with scoliosis to the challenges she faced with her family. She told them she had overcome it

> and was standing there before all of them truly happy. Selling boats doesn't matter. Being happy does."
>
> —Johnny Morris,
> founder and CEO of Bass Pro Shops

I was scared to death as I gave that speech. My chest was pounding as I walked up there, but I told myself to just be genuine and speak from the heart. I never knew exactly what part of my story inspired Johnny so much, but it seemed to inspire the people in that room, too.

The crowd at that convention rose and gave me a standing ovation. That meant a lot to me. I loved being able to impact the lives of everyday people, people who loved pool, and people who knew absolutely nothing about the sport.

It was always my mission to be an inspiration as I transcended the sport. In December 2022, when ESPN released my *30 for 30* documentary, *Jeanette Lee Vs.*, I realized I had done just that.

As I watched that documentary, I heard words about me that made me blush, and made me smile, and made me cry.

"Face it America. You only watch pool because of Jeanette Lee. If someone thinks of the word pool, they visualize Jeanette Lee."

"Jeanette is powerful. On the table, she will eat you alive. The tongues that would hang out with Jeanette? Yes, yes, yes. She was on fire."

"She embodied how women have come to their own in one of the most decidedly male institutions."

"She's had a lot of struggles. Climbed every mountain and got to the very top. It's an amazing story."

I did climb to the top. And when I was there, I had fans waiting around every corner. And it was the fans who lifted me up, years later, when cancer came to destroy me, and I hit my rock bottom.

CHAPTER 18

MAYBE CANCER HADN'T DESTROYED THE BLACK WIDOW AFTER ALL

STAGE 4 OVARIAN CANCER was swirling inside my body like an out-of-control tornado in January 2021, leaving deadly cells in its wake.

And there was absolutely nothing I could do about it. I couldn't do what I had always done to overcome my weaknesses or my opponents. I couldn't practice terminal cancer away. I couldn't strike this disease with a cue and make it fall deep into a corner pocket, never to be seen again. I couldn't wear a big, clunky brace to keep it at bay like I did with my scoliosis.

And I couldn't sweet talk this ugly disease into doing what I desperately wanted it to do, get the hell out of my body.

Instead, I would have to be pumped with drugs that, in all reality, were nothing more than poison coursing through my veins. I would have to go through intense pain, nausea, depression, unthinkable fatigue, and deep fear. Then, I would have to wait.

Would the treatments even work? The statistics, the odds, and the opinions of the medical journals, were all against me. I would have to pray for a miracle, an intervention from God that would let me live.

It's hard to explain the depth of loneliness that overcomes your soul when you start pondering your own mortality and thinking about all the things you will miss.

Your daughters' sweet hugs, their weddings, and your grandchildren. The feeling of the ocean waves splashing on your face. The thrill of winning a game of pool against a really good opponent. Gathering with your family for a home-cooked meal that sends a warm rush throughout your body. The amazement that washes over you as fans show their adoration.

There are so many beautiful things in this world to miss.

It's heart-wrenching to think about what will happen after you're gone from this Earth. Your daughters trying desperately to be brave, and sobbing, after they've watched their mother take her last breath. Your parents standing over your casket at the funeral, and sobbing. Your sister giving your eulogy, and sobbing.

You will be gone, but the magic of the world will carry on. The roses will still bloom, the warm rain will still sprinkle, and the sun will still set, showing off God's creativity in a different way every single night.

But you won't be there to see any of it, and that is an incredibly devastating reality to ponder.

In the early days of my diagnosis, I told only a few people that I had cancer, just family and a few close friends.

The first night I came home from the hospital, the only people who knew of my diagnosis were my pool mentor, Gene Nagy; my boyfriend, Gene Allen; my longtime friend Julie, who was living with me as my nanny; and my dear friend Mark Wilson, who happened to be visiting at the time for the New Year's holiday.

When I walked into my house, I told my daughters that I'd had a bad reaction to a new medication. It was just an excuse so I didn't have to tell them what was really going on. Cancer.

They were so happy to see me. We ate dinner together and then I watched them as they laughed in the living room watching TV. *How can I tell them?* I thought to myself. *Will this be the last time I see them laugh like this again?*

I went to bed that night and stared at the ceiling. I couldn't sleep. My heart was so heavy that I almost couldn't breathe. I knew I would have to tell my mom and my sister, but I couldn't yet. I wasn't sure I could get the words out to them.

Instead, I got out of bed and walked over to my home office, curled up in my recliner, and I called Janet Atwell. Janet was a dear friend and a breast cancer survivor. I remember being at a tournament with Janet in Michigan during her cancer fight. She had on a cap, but no wig. I remember thinking how courageous she was. Janet was, and still is, my role model.

On the phone that night, I called Janet. "I have cancer. It's really bad." I cried as I talked to Janet, and she listened. I told her I needed to focus. I needed to make sure my three daughters would be okay.

The only thing I could think about after I heard the words, "Stage 4 cancer," were Cheyenne, Chloe, and Savannah.

> "Jeanette was not just worried about leaving her daughters without a mom, but she was also worried about being broke, leaving them with no financial security. That weighed heaviest on her heart."
>
> —Tom George, Lee's longtime manager

I was in a very dark place when I called Tom days after my diagnosis. Of course, I wanted to talk to him about the cancer but, mostly,

I told him how worried I was that I might not leave my daughters with enough money before they get established in adulthood.

The COVID-19 pandemic had wreaked havoc on my Tampa Bay APA pool league and taken away my bread and butter, making public appearances. The WPBA tournaments had all but disappeared and so had my sponsorships.

The pandemic was raging everywhere, taking the lives of people with *healthy* immune systems. I now had two autoimmune diseases, and was incredibly worried all the time.

Those months were obviously harsh emotionally, reeling from a terminal diagnosis, but in some ways they were even more harsh financially. I went from making a pretty good living to making practically nothing within a matter of months. If it wasn't for APA choosing to continue to pay me as their national spokesperson, I'm not sure how we would have survived.

When I would force myself to check my bank account balance, I hated the numbers I saw. My whole life seemed to be imploding in front of my eyes.

After my phone call with Tom, he immediately packed up his car and drove from his home in Atlanta to Tampa. He had talked to my longtime doctor, Don Wardell, who told him, "Tom, whatever you're going to do, you better hurry. Three, maybe four months, is not unreasonable."

My life, at that time, was being measured in months, weeks, and days.

When Tom arrived at my home, I quickly realized he wasn't there for small talk or to coddle me. He was there to do business, to help me. Tom brought up the idea of starting a GoFundMe campaign. That was a hard "no" for me.

I wasn't the type to ever ask for help. I always wanted to do things on my own, and just because I had cancer, that didn't mean I would start asking people for handouts now. Why? Because, quite honestly,

I didn't feel like my story was any more special than anyone else's story. Wasn't everyone in America hurting right now?

Plus, there was my pride. I had made so much money and, yes, I had let a lot of money fall through my hands, but I don't regret the things I invested in. I invested in helping others. I spent a lot of money doing things for other people, and I'd do it all over again.

That, coupled with me having multiple major surgeries in which I was uninsured, made it difficult to save a lot. I never imagined I would stop playing pool so early. Now I feel dumb for not expecting it, with my medical history.

I had such a bad medical history that it was impossible for me to get medical coverage until Obamacare. I went through an awful divorce and I was just learning a new business (Tampa Bay APA), while raising three girls as a single mom. I had no close friends or family in Tampa. I invested in buying a business because I knew there would come a day when I couldn't compete all the time and I didn't want to wait until then to buy a business. Why not buy a business while you're still hot and making better income. Yet, just a few years later, everything went away at once.

As I talked to Tom about all of that, still insisting a GoFundMe campaign wasn't how to solve my financial struggles, the genius marketer in him came out.

Tom is good at laying things out straight, and he is brilliant at convincing people to do things they might not want to do. Tom kept talking and talking and talking, and he kept pleading with me. "Now is not the time for false pride, Jeanette," he said. "You're dying."

A GoFundMe campaign made sense, Tom said, because I had equity. I had no idea, at first, what in the world he was talking about.

But Tom went on, and he told me I had built up equity by the way I had treated people throughout my career. The power of my personality, the late nights I had stayed to play pool with random fans, not leaving until I had signed every single autograph. The charity appearances I had made, the way I mentored young people—the way I had lived my life.

> "When Jeanette was interacting with her fans, they hadn't just *met* Jeanette Lee. They thought they *knew* Jeanette Lee. There was a connection. She didn't really know them. She couldn't possibly remember all their names, but they got the impression that she knew them. And that was a beautiful thing."
>
> —Tom George, Lee's longtime manager

I always wanted to be humble and approachable. That was intentional on my part. I wanted people to feel like they had a chance, not with me, but in life. When I met those fans, I wanted them to see me, talk with me, and believe that they could reach their dreams, too. No matter what they had gone through, or what they were facing, they could persevere.

As we talked on Tom's visit to Tampa, he told me, if done right, we could use that equity I had built up to help my daughters, to make sure they were secure, and that they would be okay should the unthinkable odds I was facing become reality, and I died.

I finally agreed to the GoFundMe campaign for one reason, actually three reasons: my three sweet, precious daughters.

Tom quickly began his marketing magic. Setting up the fundraising site was easy, but he had to make sure people knew about it, to make sure it caught fire. That meant timing the launch of the campaign with the announcement of my terminal diagnosis. The world would learn for the first time that I had Stage 4 ovarian cancer.

The billiards community and press jumped on the story immediately, in full force. First, the big players like Mike Panozzo at *Billiards Digest*, Mike Howerton at *AZ Billiards*, and the American Poolplayers

Association, posted the news. Quickly, the smaller pool publications picked up my story, too.

My marketing agency, Octagon, deserves major credit. In 2021, I wasn't making them any money, but all those people there stopped what they were doing to help me.

Teddy Bloch, who at the time was the director of sales and marketing, came up with a plan to make sure the news of my cancer diagnosis reached the entire world. And Alyssa Romano, vice president of communications, pushed my story out to all the big names in sports media. None of this was going to make Octagon a penny.

> "We owe this to Jeanette. She's been such a great client. This is the right thing to do."
>
> —Phil de Picciotto,
> president of Octagon, March 2021

The Asian Hall of Fame was incredible to me, too. I was one of their inductees, alongside other notable Asians like architect I.M. Pei, martial artist and actor Bruce Lee, and NFL defensive tackle Manu Tuiasosopo.

The hall of fame's push, led by its president and CEO Maki Hsieh, who is one of my biggest heroes, resulted in hundreds of articles being written about me in China, Hong Kong, Singapore, India, and the Philippines.

Along with the news of my cancer, all those articles mentioned my GoFundMe campaign.

"It is with heavy hearts that we share that our friend and billiards icon, Jeanette Lee, has been diagnosed with Stage IV ovarian cancer. The cancer has metastasized throughout her body," the GoFundMe page read in 2021. "Her prognosis is currently unknown and depends upon her body's response to the first phase of treatment she is now undergoing. Left untreated, this stage and type of cancer can be swiftly terminal."

The page went on to talk about my daughters, Cheyenne, who was 16 at the time, Chloe, 11, and Savannah, 10. "Jeanette's largest and most pressing concern is the well-being of her three young girls. Jeanette has been a single mother for the last several years. The future care, well-being, and education of her girls is the biggest cause of anxiety for her."

When the campaign launched, I had no idea what to expect, and neither did Tom, despite his reassurances at the beginning.

Tom was sitting anxiously at his desk as the GoFundMe page went live. He said he had never been so nervous about anything in his life. He had promised me this was the right thing to do. But he had been warned that the pool-playing public was notoriously tight-fisted.

That was certainly not the case.

> "I'm sitting at my desk just waiting, and then boom, boom, boom, donation after donation started pouring in. From $5, $10, and $20 donations to $50, $100, and $500 donations, and then a few major financial gifts. The love from the billiards community and beyond was immense."
>
> —Tom George, Lee's longtime manager

The original goal for my GoFundMe campaign was $100,000, but it quickly catapulted to nearly $250,000. Beyond the public campaign, there were many private donations made to help me battle cancer, rest and rejuvenate, care for my girls and their future, and allow me to spend quality time making memories with my loved ones. Those included gifts from NASCAR legend Tony Stewart, Bass Pro Shops founder Johnny Morris, and Heisman Trophy winner Reggie Bush, three of my good friends.

Glitzy benefits were held for me, without Tom or anyone else asking for them to be held, including one put on by the American Poolplayers Association and *Billiards Digest*, called "A Night to Celebrate The Black Widow."

Smaller pool halls, like Brewlands Billiards, Borderline Billiards, and Amsterdam Billiards, chipped in, holding their own fundraisers. One of them raised $3,310, not a lot of money in the whole scheme of things. But those were the fundraisers that meant the most to me. I knew that $3,310 had come from a lot of people giving what little they could afford—$5 here and $10 there. I had friends and fellow professionals, like Jeannie Seaver, Sonya Chbeeb, Jeremy and Amy Jones, Janet Atwell, Mike Immonen, Tyler Styer, Albin Ouschan, and Joshua Filler hosting fundraisers, a couple that raised well over $20,000.

Along with the donations came all the messages from fans. Some of them were cockamamie cancer cures, but most of them were really nice notes of inspiration, prayers, and memories they had with me. A lot of them brought me to tears.

There was one letter from Las Vegas, from the mother of a son with autism, who had come to an appearance of mine years before. She wrote that her son's self-esteem had been low, but as I walked him around the table, teaching him shots, she watched him come out of his shell. She wrote that her son had never forgotten his time with me.

That letter made me cry, and so did hundreds of other messages. I realized that I had made a difference in many lives.

As the love from the billiards community, and beyond, descended on me, I went from a very dark place—going through chemotherapy, sick and nauseous, worried and alone, and so scared about the future for my daughters—to seeing a beautiful ray of light.

> "Jeanette was able to find something out, something that is invaluable. She found out that she is broadly loved—broadly

> loved throughout the sports and billiards community. She didn't know it, but I knew it, and everyone else knew it."
> —Tom George, Lee's longtime manager

I took that ray of light, all those messages from fans, fellow pool players, famous people, everyday people, and old friends, and I carried them with me as I went through my treatments. They were invaluable to me.

And man, those treatments were brutal. I had been through pain before. Scoliosis is cruel. But this pain was different. It was as emotional as it was physical. I would sit in a room without windows inside a Tampa Bay cancer center for four long hours as a cocktail of drugs pumped through a port in my chest.

My body would ache, and I never knew if it was because of all my previous surgeries or because my treatments had been stopped for my two autoimmune diseases (ankylosing spondylitis and fibromyalgia) or if the pain was because of the cancer.

I always brought a lumbar support pillow to try to ease the pain and a big thermos of coffee. I packed oatmeal to take to my treatments. The doctors told me I had to keep my weight up, but that became harder every cycle of chemotherapy, because all I wanted to do was sleep.

I would have good intentions each afternoon to eat a big healthy dinner, but sometimes, by 5:00 PM, I would be so worn out I'd go to bed and sleep right through dinner. I did that a lot. To be honest, I pretty much slept through the entire months of June and July in 2021.

As my hair started to fall out from the chemo, I shaved my head, and watched my shiny black locks fall to the floor. I never wore a wig. I wanted the world to see what cancer really was. I didn't want to hide it.

I battled through the nausea, throwing up all the time, unable to eat the spicy foods I loved so much. I would lie in bed so tired, the kind of fatigue that sleep didn't help. I would get up and go to my next chemo treatment, because I am stubborn, and because I had to live for my girls.

After my third round of chemo, doctors said I needed surgery to remove my ovaries, uterus, and small masses near my abdomen. That didn't really scare me. Surgery was nothing new to me. I had been in the operating room many times before for my back, but I had never been there for an operation that would, possibly, save my life.

No matter how awful those months of treatments were for me, I knew I was blessed beyond measure. I had childhood friends, cousins, my mother, my sister, pool players—so many people there to lift me up, and make sure I was okay.

They would come to my house to make home-cooked meals, to clean the bathrooms, to be with my girls, and to do all sorts of amazing things I didn't even know I needed.

Two of my godchildren put together a binder with information and directions and tips. "Rub steroid gel on painful areas," one entry said. Another was an alert that I had choked on frozen grapes. And there were the reminder pages with photos of the various pills I had to take every morning, afternoon, and night.

My friends and family filled the dry-erase board in the entryway of my house with my upcoming doctor's appointments, because the chemo was making my brain foggy and I forgot a lot. I would be talking and stop in the middle of my sentence, not able to remember what I had been saying seconds before.

"That's the most annoying thing," I told *Sports Illustrated,* when the publication came to my home to do an article as I fought cancer, titled "The Little Blessings of The Black Widow." "I tend to be fairly articulate, and I'm worried I won't get it back.... Then it's like everything has really been taken from me. I'm just a shell. I'm still walking, but I've already lost what everyone on the planet knows me for: A world champion playing pool."

It was hard seeing my daughters watch me battle cancer, but none of it was entirely new to them. They had lived through all of my physical struggles. I had been sick most of their lives, not from cancer, but from the debilitating pain of scoliosis.

> "Some people just kind of think, 'Oh, Jeanette Lee's just this superhuman, and she's so cool,' but she still is human, and she still goes through that pain."
>
> —Savannah Breedlove, Lee's daughter

When my six cycles of chemo were over, and all those brutal chemo treatments were finished, I knew my Stage 4 ovarian cancer was gone. I wanted it to be gone. I had prayed for it to be gone. It had to be gone.

That's what I told myself in those deep, sometimes dark, moments of thought that only a person battling cancer can understand.

I had done everything I was supposed to do. But my doctor told me otherwise. Cancer didn't care that I had followed its protocol. Cancer has its own ideas. "No, you're not in remission," my doctor told me after my chemo finished in 2021. During the total hysterectomy, halfway through my chemo treatments, my oncology surgeon was not able to safely remove the lymph nodes that we believed were cancerous like she had previously planned. They told me that once they got into surgery and opened me up, they were lying in a way that they felt was not worth the risk of nicking and causing more cancer to spread. So now all we could do was pray that the ones that remained would disappear during the remaining chemo treatments. Unfortunately, in the end, they were still there.

I didn't understand the words I was hearing from my doctor. I asked and I pleaded. What would it take for me to go into remission? I'll never forget my doctor's words:

"I'm sorry, Jeanette, but I don't believe you're ever going to go into remission."

They were going to put me on maintenance chemo pills for the rest of my life. I also learned from them that unfortunately ovarian cancer was a type of cancer that almost always comes back. Imagine being told that when you thought you'd done everything right. Sadly, unlike some other cancers, there was still no cure.

I was devastated. I felt like I was standing on the edge of a cliff, and that I would be standing on that cliff for the rest of my life, just waiting for that little shove that would push me over the edge into the darkness, into death.

My family was devastated, too.

> "I automatically thought Jeanette would live longer than [me]. Now, in some ways, we're competing."
>
> —Sonja Lee, Jeanette's mother

I brushed away my mother's sadness and the never-in-remission talk from doctors, and I forged ahead. Now that the worst chemo was over, I wanted to move on, get stronger, live my life again. I wanted to forget that ovarian cancer is known for returning.

But my body had other plans. I was still in too much pain and my nausea wouldn't go away. I was always so tired and I was heavily medicated. I found it hard to think, analyze, make plans, or remember simple things. I started going to physical therapy and had to face how *severely* my muscles had atrophied. I was losing weight, had no strength, and it felt like getting my fit body back was going to be impossible. My depression worsened.

I wanted so badly to push through, though. I wanted to keep sharing my journey with the world. I was always looking for ways I could make something good come out of all the crap that happened to me. I wanted to give people hope and inspire them to join my journey on the road to recovery. I knew I was not alone and I wanted others like me to know that too. There were tens of thousands of fans following me. My point was that, although we sometimes can't help the things that happen to us, when we're victimized, we don't have to stay a victim. If you get knocked down, rest, recover, but don't stay there forever. Never give up on yourself, on your plan for a better life. If you give up, you're guaranteeing that nothing will ever get better for you. It can only get worse. Love yourself enough to be strong, even when you don't feel strong.

I felt a responsibility to stay authentic, never give up, and do it publicly. But deep inside I was hurting and scared. Don't get me wrong. I still intended to beat it. I still believed that God had and has a greater plan for me and I wasn't meant to die right then from cancer. But getting out of bed excited to start my day had slowed down. I was tired and sad. I found myself in bed way too much, which only made me feel worse about myself. I have a responsibility to my girls, after all. I wanted to be stronger and be someone they could be proud of, but my body and mind always seemed to have other ideas.

Thankfully, I have great friends.

My partners, Anthony and Stephanie, were doing a great job running the league. That took a ton of pressure off of me. They were always stopping by to drop off some food, or just visit. Jeannie Seaver and Sonya Chbeeb, who used to visit often to eat dinner together or maybe even play a little pool, were calling me or coming by every week. One day, they invited me to ride with them to the Inaugural Omega's Diamond Open Tournament in Aiken, South Carolina. Because of COVID and my condition, flying wasn't an option. But I could get out of the house, ride, and room with them. They would keep me safe and help in any way. Jeannie was also a nurse in the oncology field. I considered the offer for a moment.

"Yes! I'd love to!"

Maybe this was what I needed. To get out of the house, go play pool, and surround myself with people just like me who loved the game. I had been getting so many kind and supportive messages and all kinds of donations from my pool community. I thought that it would be great to be seen in public, to be seen still fighting the good fight. Plus, I wanted them all to know how thankful I was. I hopped in the car and made my first appearance since I had my cancer diagnosis eight months before.

Because of all my treatments, I had not been able to practice for that tournament. I didn't care. I wanted to experience that feeling again, to play at a green felt table, to connect with the fans who had supported me. I wanted to be out there among them.

I had no idea how well I would play in that tournament, but I knew I would give it everything I had. I just wanted to feel normal again.

Inside a warehouse that had been converted into a pool hall, next to a little hair salon in the uppercase Deep South, 20 miles from Augusta, Georgia, Marianne Raulerson, the tournament director, started crying when I walked in.

"I cannot believe Jeanette Lee is at my tournament," she sobbed, mostly tears of happiness that I was okay.

Allison Fisher was there, too. Now Allison had been my archnemesis throughout most of my career. While she and I were competing, we were friendly and polite, but I would hardly call us friends. But when she saw me, she walked toward me with tears in her eyes. She hugged me. She said she was heartbroken to hear the news and that she wished the best for me. Then she proceeded to tell me that she couldn't believe how strong and brave I was being, that what I was doing—sharing my cancer journey with the world to help people—took so much courage. I was genuinely touched and thankful. She didn't have to go out of her way to say that to me.

A couple days later, I drew Allison in the tournament, and the match was going to be streamed live. When I got there to play, she greeted me and hugged me again. This time, we held each other for a couple minutes. It was a very special moment for me. She had come to our match dressed in one of my Black Widow jerseys. What an honoring, caring, and humble thing to do. With all the egos that come with being a world-caliber champion, I'd never seen or imagined any male or female top pro playing in a match wearing someone else's jersey. That was incredibly special.

All these years later, the WPBA women seemed to be coming together. Maybe all my top peers didn't still hate me. Marianne, Jeannie, and Sonya encouraged me to bring all my merch because the fans would love it and I could make a little money. But I never expected Allison and so many of the other top male and female players—really, superstars in our world—to go to the booth to buy and wear my jersey all throughout the tournament. I'd always offered pros a discount if they wanted to buy one for a friend or family member, but this time, Allison and all the other players refused the discount. I can't tell you how incredible that felt. I'll never forget it.

> "You don't wish that on anyone. [Jeanette and I have had our] things over the years, but I think we've been around each other for so long, you know? You're like a big family in a way."
>
> —Allison Fisher,
> billiards hall of famer, in ESPN's *Jeanette Lee Vs.*

Up to that tournament, I had never finished out of the money in a pro tournament. I had always placed high enough to take home a part of the winnings, sometimes thousands of dollars, sometimes a few hundred.

And it was no different that day. Eight months after my cancer diagnosis, I had somehow, magically, finished seventh, high enough for the money. The only two players I lost to at that tournament were the finalists, pros Allison Fisher and Kristina Tkach. I didn't go into that tournament thinking I was going to win. It had been years since I trained for a tournament. This was only to get out and be seen by the public who had rallied behind me during my fight, to give back to pool, and to be around my old scene. I was right: competing did give me comfort and encouragement. I didn't have any expectations on how I'd play. To my surprise, I didn't play all that badly.

Despite everything against me, I had kept my streak alive. My life, it seemed, was finally looking up. Maybe it was time for goodness to prevail and for me to finally start to heal. Maybe everything was going to be okay.

But as always seems to happen in my life, evil returned, this time in a different form. Three months after that tournament in South Carolina, I took a fall that sent me spiraling toward rock bottom and left me more scared than I had ever been in my life.

It was December 15, 2021, when I started my trek to New York City in my boyfriend's motor home. I was headed on the month-long trip of a lifetime.

When I found out I was facing terminal cancer, I started talking to my sister, Doris, who lives in Hong Kong. We crafted a plan to travel to New York to visit all the places where we grew up, to spend some time together and to visit old friends and family, people that we hadn't seen in a very long time.

On the ride there in my RV, I walked up to the front to talk to my then-boyfriend, Gene, who was driving. I shouldn't have. I always had a very, very strict rule with my daughters, and anyone else inside the motor home. Never get up when the vehicle is in motion, unless it's absolutely necessary.

About the time I made it to the front of the RV to talk to Gene, an oncoming car veered into our lane. When Gene slammed on the brakes to avoid hitting the car, I was thrown backward, flipped over, and I fell headfirst down the steep stairwell of this massive 39-foot motor home. It was not good.

My fall was not like a normal person falling. Because of my scoliosis, my entire back is fused. Most people's bodies would have crumbled down the stairs. I fell like a plank, like a piece of wood, no way to protect myself.

I was rushed to the emergency room, where scans and MRIs ruled out anything serious. I was released and told to follow up with my doctor when I returned home from my trip.

But once we made it to my cousin Esther's home in New York, I suddenly took a very bad turn. Something was seriously wrong. All kinds of scary, weird symptoms converged on me all at once. I was having a hard time talking. I knew what I wanted to say, but the words wouldn't come out.

I was dizzy and off-balance. I fell three times. I was clumsy. Whatever I tried to put in my hand, I could not grasp. I was dropping things all the time, dropping a fork, dropping a cup, dropping a pen, dropping my cane.

I was having difficulty thinking, my speech was worsening, I was extremely fatigued, and I was in pain. It was brutal. It was incredibly scary, because I had no idea what this was. What if it was the cancer spreading even further? What if I was nearing the end?

I went back to the emergency room, where more tests were done. Doctors diagnosed me with severe spinal stenosis—a narrowing of the spaces within the spine which can put pressure on nerves that travel through the spine. The stenosis was the cause of the weakness, imbalance, and the pain I was enduring.

I was scheduled for emergency laminectomy surgery for my cauda equina and spinal stenosis, the second surgery in one year that would possibly save my life.

Ten days after surgery, I felt well enough to sit up in my hospital bed in Stony Brook, New York, and stream a Facebook video. More than 180,000 people hung on my every word as I updated them on my health battles.

I told them that January 2022 had been a rough start for a New Year, but not nearly as rough as the start of 2021, when the cancer had come for me. I talked about how I hated the way my hair was growing back in sparse patches, but how I knew that wasn't anything to dwell on. My blessings were what I should focus on.

"I'm so thankful for having incredible family and friends, and the support system that has been out there, and all my fans out there who have also been sending prayers—all that matters," I said. "Just look up, look forward to the day, look forward to tomorrow, and see what you can make of it."

I talked and I smiled in that video, but underneath the façade, I knew the odds were not good for Stage 4 ovarian cancer. But I also felt like if I went by the odds, I never would have become a world champion, and so I wasn't going to go with the odds this time, either.

Weeks after I shot that Facebook video from my hospital bed, I was walking around New York City with a cane, as a film crew from ESPN recorded me in Brooklyn and Long Island. The network was there to do a *30 for 30* documentary on me, titled *Jeanette Lee Vs.*

Maybe cancer hadn't destroyed The Black Widow, after all.

> "Jeanette battled fierce opponents, trying times, debilitating pain, personal demons, and persistent criticism, but she remains a singular presence from a breakout era of pool—an unforgettable figure, The Black Widow."
>
> —Ursula Liang, director of *Jeanette Lee Vs.*

Even with a terminal cancer diagnosis, The Black Widow seemed to be alive and well. ESPN was still following me, and the network wanted to tell the world my story.

The story of a girl who fell in love with pool at exactly the right time.

CHAPTER 19

FALLING IN LOVE WITH POOL AT EXACTLY THE RIGHT TIME

I WAS 15 YEARS OLD when I fell in love with a blond-haired, teenage pool player with piercing blue eyes. He would wrap his arm around my waist, give me a kiss, and bend over the table for his next shot.

Greg was my first love, a guy I met on the school bus when I was going to The Bronx High School of Science. He was dreamy. He had eyelashes that went on for days and I fawned over them. He was absolutely perfect, a badass, who was also sweet, and a little bit shy.

Greg and I fell hard for one another, that kind of mysterious, giddy, butterflies-in-the-stomach, first-time love. We would cut classes at Bronx Science to make out and play pool. Greg would hover behind my body at the table, teach me how to break a rack, and hold a cue.

When we were hanging out with his friends, we'd smoke pot, drink tequila, and then sneak off to his parents' summer home on Fire

Island to be together without our parents around. I loved everything about Greg, but I never really liked pot. It made me sleepy and paranoid. I could only handle a few drags. There were a few times I smoked more, and that was scary. I didn't like the feeling of not having my wits about me.

When Greg and I hung out alone, we never smoked weed. But if I was hanging out with him and his guy friends, I definitely felt pressure to do it. The guys never pressured me but, in my mind, I needed to smoke to fit in and seem cool.

My favorite memories with Greg were at the pool halls he took me to. He introduced me to this game I knew nothing about and, as I watched him play, I loved everything about it.

I didn't really love the atmosphere of the pool halls we played in. They were dark and smoky, a place I knew my mother would have hated. But I didn't care about any of that. I was smitten with Greg.

Throughout my career, people have always asked me when I started playing pool, and I struggle with that question. The first time I picked up a cue was with Greg, but that's not when my obsession was born.

When I played pool with Greg, I fell in love with the idea that billiards might be a sport I could actually play. And there were very few sports I could play. Until then, I hadn't been competitive in anything, except card games, since my scoliosis surgery at 13.

As a little girl, I had always been competitive. I always wanted to be the best. I always wanted to rule the backyard of my apartment building and beat the guys. But as I grew older, the scoliosis slowed me down. That evil curve in my spine always tried to stop me.

When I played pool with Greg, I didn't feel that pain. The game was a slow-paced, easy-going sport, and it didn't hurt my back. Of course, a few years later, I learned that pool was very hard on my back, when I played it hour after hour, day after day, match after match.

But at the time, I just loved Greg and, so, I loved pool.

So I guess I started playing pool with Greg when I was 15 years old but, in my mind, that isn't when I *really* started playing pool, really practicing and focusing on the sport.

I didn't *really* start playing pool until I was 18 and I walked into Chelsea Billiards, became obsessed, and then, somehow, in an unexpected twist of fate, became a star. I owe part of my success to timing, which is everything—being in the right place at the right time.

When I walked into Chelsea Billiards in 1989, a pool frenzy was sweeping the nation, brought on by Tom Cruise and Paul Newman, who had invaded the silver screen in theaters three years before with the box office smash hit film *The Color of Money*. It was the sequel to *The Hustler*, starring Jackie Gleason and Newman.

The Hustler is my absolute favorite pool movie. I've watched it more times than I can count, and I get chills every time.

Without that movie, which led to *The Color of Money*, I'm not sure I could have ever become a superstar in the sport. That movie awakened a dormant billiards industry in the 1980s.

> "So many people saw that movie and were kind of blown away by it."
>
> —R.A. "Jake" Dyer,
> pool historian and author
> of *The Hustler & The Champ*

Pool became all the rage in the late '80s. It went from a sport played in cheap joints by blue-collar workers with cigarettes hanging out of their mouths, munching on nachos in between shots, to a glamorous sport for celebrities and rich people. *The Color of Money* turned pool into a yuppie craze.

The dank and dingy billiards halls with linoleum floors inside that had flashing neon signs outside started to fade away, replaced by posh, carpeted, upscale halls frequented by men with slicked-back hair, wearing three-piece suits, with glamorous women on their arms.

Mansions in California, flashy resorts lining the coasts, and five-star hotels started moving green felt tables into their midst. High-end pool halls began to spring up all over the country. Two years after the premier of *The Color of Money*, the number of pool rooms in America had increased 400 percent.

As I began my career playing at one of those new, glitzy halls named Chelsea Billiards, pool had catapulted to one of the top 10 participation sports played in the U.S.

Gallup estimated that 33 million Americans were pool players, ranked billiards fourth among games played by men, and reported that the percentage of all players had grown by 430 percent since 1959.

As I bet men $5, $10, or $20 a game at New York City tables, the industry was exploding. A staggering $500 million was being spent on the game annually. Equipment sales increased more than 100 percent after *The Color of Money* was released, according to a survey by the Billiard Congress of America, which represents manufacturers, retailers, and players.

I made my debut at the height of a pool renaissance, which was nothing more than pure luck. Pool, after all, wasn't always a sport that could produce superstars like The Black Widow.

> "Billiards has always gone through cycles. You are dealing with a game that goes back centuries. Washington and Jefferson were players, and Mark Twain made it a part of *Every Man's Education*."
>
> —Paul Roberts,
> Billiard Congress of America,
> *Los Angeles Times*, 1988

Pool got its first modern day revival in 1961 when the movie *The Hustler* was released. In case you haven't seen it, *The Hustler* stars Paul Newman as "Fast Eddie" Felson, a small-time pool hustler who challenges legendary, real-life pool icon Minnesota Fats, played by Jackie Gleason.

America fell in love with the sport of pool, mostly, because of the hustling in the movie. The idea of being able to win with wits, not just skill at the table, lured them in.

For me, pool was always about the skill of the game, but I always knew that wasn't how most novice players saw the game.

A year after *The Hustler* was released, *The Music Man* came onto the silver screen, a movie that characterized the local pool hall as a place for gambling, hustling, swearing, and drinking. It captivated audiences nationwide.

The Music Man had debuted on stage as one of the most popular musicals of all time in 1957. One of the songs from the show, called "Ya Got Trouble," belted out the lyrics: "You got trouble, folks, right here in River City, trouble with a capital 'T'; And that rhymes with 'P' and that stands for pool."

Hollywood made pool sexy in the 1960s and that made Minnesota Fats famous. As my manager Tom George always says, "The American sports public only has enough room in their collective memory bank for one pool player a generation."

Before me, that generational player was Minnesota Fats, who was born Rudolf Walter Wanderone in New York City in 1913. He got his start playing pool as a young boy and, by the time he was a teenager, he was a traveling pool hustler. During World War II, he went around the country hustling servicemen.

Wanderone was a heavy set, Swiss-American, pro billiards player who never won a major pool tournament, but he was the most recognized name in billiards. He wasn't just a player. He was an entertainer, and he was a fierce advocate for the sport. Wanderone was even inducted into the Billiard Congress of America Hall of Fame in 1984 for his decades-long promotion of the sport.

At exactly the same time Minnesota Fats was making his name, Willie Mosconi was on the pool scene, too. Mosconi is widely considered one of the greatest pool players of all time, winning the World Straight Pool Championship 15 times between 1941 and 1957. But outside of billiards circles, most people don't know Mosconi's name. They do know Minnesota Fats' name.

> "Jeanette became the Minnesota Fats of her generation, that one player of the 1990s and 2000s. And today, she is still the only generational pool player whose name is widely recognized outside of the sport."
>
> —Tom George, Lee's longtime manager

How and when and who exactly brought billiards to the United States has never really been determined.

Most likely, Dutch and English settlers brought the game to the states, according to the Billiard Congress of America. It was in the 1700s that American cabinet makers began to build exquisite, lavish billiard tables.

The sport soon spread throughout the colonies, among the rich and the poor. Future president George Washington was reported to have won a match in 1748 at the age of 18. By 1830, public rooms devoted entirely to billiards began to appear. The most famous was Bassford's, a New York room that catered to stockbrokers.

From there, the father of American billiards stepped in. His name was Michael Phelan, an immigrant from Ireland who, in 1850, wrote the first American book on the game. Phelan is credited with the incredible rise in popularity of pool in the U.S. during the 19th century.

As a relentless advocate for pocket billiards, Phelan devised rules and set standards of behavior. He added diamonds to the table to assist in aiming, and he developed new table and cushion designs. Phelan was also the first American billiard columnist for *Leslie's Illustrated Weekly*.

With Phelan leading the way, the sport of billiards took off, and its popularity soared. And then its popularity petered out. And then it took off again. And then it petered out again.

> "At the turn of the century, it was a gentleman's game. In the '30s, it was a Depression pastime, and there was a love-hate, romantic rogue appeal attached to it. It always seemed that over the course of decades, it could be huge, and the next minute it's out."
>
> —Paul Roberts,
> Billiard Congress of America,
> *Los Angeles Times*, 1988

I was lucky enough to come onto the pool scene when the sport was booming. I have to thank my teenage boyfriend, Greg, for introducing me to the sport and inspiring a curiosity that would later draw me to Chelsea Billiards.

I never got to thank Greg for that. Until my cancer diagnosis, I hadn't talked to Greg since I moved to the West Coast for my professional pool career at the age of 21. But I always thought of him and wondered what became of him.

When my cancer became public nearly three decades later, Greg's wife reached out to me. She told me he wanted to talk to me. Of course, I said yes. Of course, I wanted to talk to Greg.

In my life, there have been only a few guys I have really fallen for since Greg, but, even then, I never felt the kind of love that I had with him. Maybe that was because we were so young and free, and he was my first true love.

On our phone call, Greg was so nice to me. He told me he only wanted the best for me and that he was so sorry I had cancer. It was wonderful to talk with him. It was emotional, and it was a bit of closure.

Greg and I had been so in love in high school, but our parents had always tried to keep us apart. They didn't think we were good for one another, probably because we were always hanging out, smoking weed, doing ungodly things, and ignoring their rules.

We were deeply bonded in a forbidden love, and that made things even more titillating.

But as we got older, and as I started trying to make pool a career, Greg and I began to go down very different paths. Our relationship was shaky a lot of the time. It seemed like it was always on again, off again.

During one of our "on again" times, I went through one of the most traumatizing things I have ever been through. It was a car accident that, had things turned out differently, could have killed me.

It was late one night, when Greg picked me up from a pool room after a long, intense night of practicing. I was ready to relax and spend some time with Greg. As we headed down the Brooklyn-Queens Expressway, we had no idea that storms were coming.

But as we drove, the rain that was sprinkling quickly turned into an all-out torrent. We couldn't see anything in front of us, not even the rear lights of the cars ahead of us.

It was one of those storms that was so strong, most people would pull their cars off to the side of the road. We were in the middle of a major highway and there was no way to pull off. I was terrified.

As we were coming around a curve, I felt this really hard thump, this hit that I still can't explain to this day. It felt like we had been hammered by a monstrous dump truck. Our car had slammed into two other cars that collided in front of us.

I started screaming and sobbing, which made Greg really worried that I had been badly hurt. He started trying to comfort me, trying to make sure I was okay, trying to make sure that I hadn't been injured. I didn't care about that at the time. All I wanted to do was get out of that car.

We were stranded in the middle of the expressway and I just knew another hit was coming from behind. Greg took off his seatbelt, and he tried to grab me and pull me out on his side. He was on the safe side near the median. I was on the side with the traffic. He unhooked my seatbelt.

"Oh my God, Greg, what are we going to do?" I said to him. "We have to get out of here."

I had barely gotten those words out of my mouth when boom, we were hit again. Then we were hit again, and again. This time, it was a six-car crash. I started to panic. Without my seatbelt on I was being thrown all over the inside of the car.

Here we were, just a couple of kids, 20 years old, and all we wanted to do was get out of there, but we were wedged between cars on either side of us. Someone must have called 911. But it seemed like it took forever for the ambulance to arrive. I remember being dragged out of the car in really bad shape.

Greg and I were taken to the hospital. He had a broken leg, and that accident took my back pain to another level. And it took my emotional suffering to an extreme. It took me forever to be able to get into a car again. And storms still, to this day, scare me to death. That accident traumatized me.

I left the hospital and I went home to be with my parents, but I had severe post-traumatic stress disorder. My mom took me to stay with a Christian family on a farm retreat where people could recover from trauma and tragedy in their lives.

Even after I was better and able to get into a car, my fear of storms invaded my whole being. I remember being at Howard Beach

Billiard Club, which was located on the second floor of a building, surrounded by glass windows.

There were nights I would be there playing pool, and it would start storming. The lightning would flash and the thunder would roar and the rain would pound the windows. I could see all of it. I could hear all of it and there were times I just couldn't take it. There were many times I would break down in tears and curl up like a baby in the fetal position under the pool table. Sometimes I would literally crawl on all fours over to the jukebox and try to hide behind the machine, underneath the wires. I would try to get the sound of the music blaring from the jukebox to drown out the storm.

After that car accident, Greg and I didn't see each other for a long time. When we finally did, it was clear that our beautiful love that had blossomed at those seedy pool halls had withered away. Our relationship gradually tapered off and, eventually, ended.

To be honest, things didn't end well between Greg and me. As I began to travel, and turned pro, our paths started to veer in different directions. Neither of us agree, to this day, why we broke up. That doesn't matter now.

I am grateful to Greg for making me feel beautiful when I didn't feel beautiful, for loving me when I didn't feel like I should be loved, and for introducing me to the game of pool at exactly the right time.

And years later, as I rose to the top of the sport, I fell in love with another dreamy pool player. This time, that pool player would become my husband.

CHAPTER 20

BEING THE WIFE OF THE FLAME THROWER

I WAS 23 YEARS OLD and just beginning a relationship with a former L.A. Lakers player when George Breedlove stole my heart. George couldn't dunk a basketball or swish a three-pointer, but he could destroy just about anyone on a green felt table.

George was known on the men's professional pool circuit as "The Flame Thrower," an intense, fiery opponent who had one of the most powerful breaks of any billiards player in the world. He was confident, strong under pressure, had great fundamentals, and a sweet stroke.

He was also handsome, charming, and sexy, all in an understated kind of way. He hated being in the spotlight. He didn't like attention.

I was living in L.A. in June 1995 when I met George at a pro tournament at the Bicycle Club Casino in Bell Gardens, which was 10 miles from my home. I had a contract as the spokesperson for the club, which paid me $5,000 a month to go to their special events and mingle with the high rollers, mostly Asian men.

The Bicycle Club also ran pool tournaments, women's and men's pro events, and George happened to be at the club for one of those events. But so was a tall, dark, and handsome former Lakers player who was paired with me for a game of pool. Sparks flew.

The club held a Celebrity Pro-Am event a day or two before the pro tournament began, inviting a group of well-known people from all walks of life—famous athletes, renowned journalists, actors, and millionaire businessmen—to partner with one of the pros. Sponsors would pay to bring in the celebrities, and the media would descend on the club to cover the event.

I was chosen as one of the pros to play with a billiards amateur, though I didn't know who it would be. As I waited for the Pro-Am to begin, I saw a little girl sitting by herself and I started playing with her. I always gravitated toward kids. I always desperately wanted to be a mother.

Soon, I was called away to the room next door to start the tournament, to be matched up with my celebrity. I gave that little girl a hug and told her I had to go. Unbeknownst to me, her father had been watching us the entire time.

And her father just so happened to be the celebrity I was matched with that day, the former Lakers player. More than the way I played pool, he was impressed with how kind I was with his daughter. After we finished our Scotch Doubles match in the Pro-Am, after he had watched me shoot the lights out, he asked me for a date.

I was impressed by him, too, not necessarily his pool playing, but the way he doted on his daughter, and he was so dreamy. I said yes.

But that romance with the tall, dark, handsome NBA player would be a very short-lived romance. Very, very short. I was about to have dinner with George.

As the men's pro tournament played out at the Bicycle Club, me and my closest WPBA friend, fellow billiards champion Helena

Thornfeldt, stopped by. I was the No. 1 women's pool player in the world at the time, so I knew most of the pros.

But I didn't really know George. I had met him the year before at an event, very briefly. We were acquaintances at best. I only really *knew of* George. At that point, he was ranked sixth in the world by the men's Pro Billiards Tour.

As the tournament played out during the day, a group of the pool players, including George, made plans to go out to dinner that night. They asked me to join them, but I couldn't go. I was supposed to go on that date with the Lakers player.

But as dinner time came, my date was still working. He called me and he told me if I didn't hear from him by 7:00 PM to scrap our plans for that night and we would do something the next day.

By the time 7:00 PM came and went, I was starving, so I decided to go to dinner with the pool players. I was the only woman of the group heading to dinner with George; a couple of other pros, Tommy Kennedy and John Ditoro; and a friend, Mike Geffner, who was a sportswriter for *Billiards Digest.*

At that dinner, George was so funny and smart and sweet and cool and interesting. The only way I can describe what happened that night is "we just clicked." There was just something about George Breedlove.

After dinner, we went back to George and his friend Tommy Kennedy's shared hotel room. We watched *The Sandlot*, a movie about a group of young baseball players, set in the summer of 1962. I had never seen the movie before. That wasn't unusual. I hadn't seen many movies.

Believe it or not, even at 23 years old, I could count on one hand the movies I'd seen on the big screen. And I'd only watched maybe a dozen on television. I had, after all, been obsessed with pool since I was 18. There was never a good reason, in my mind, to waste two and a half hours on a movie when I could be playing pool. If my back went out and I did have time to watch TV, I'd rather watch pool and study the game.

But I loved *The Sandlot*. I'm pretty sure I loved that movie because George was sitting next to me. I went home that night almost giddy. I could not believe I had met a Christian pool player that was good looking, amazing at billiards, and owned his own outdoor furniture business.

Almost all the other top pros didn't have side jobs, but that also meant they didn't make a steady income. George had a steady income. I completely forgot about my plans the next day with that NBA player.

Instead, George and I hung out the next day, and the day after that. On our third date, five days after we met, we started talking about things people don't usually talk about on the third date—our future careers, how many children we would want to have, our deepest secrets, and our darkest fears.

Then, completely unexpectedly, George turned to me and said, "What if we were to get married?" That sounded good to me.

I might have only known George for five days, but I was absolutely crazy about him. He was an amazing kisser, and I so respected his faith. He was always reading the Bible and books by Christian author John MacArthur. I felt an immediate connection to George.

The one thing that had always been missing in my past relationships, the one thing that I had never shared with a man, was my faith in God. I remember thinking, "Could this guy be any more perfect?"

When George and I became engaged after such a short time, my family—and just about everyone who knew me—frowned upon the idea. But I was enamored with the way George played pool. I liked that he was so genuine, seemed so kind, and was funny and smart.

A few weeks later, I realized that saying "yes" to George was the best decision of my life. Not only did I love George, but—unlike that smooth-talking, Porsche-driving Lakers player, whose eyes were as dreamy as they came—George was a down-to-earth, faith-driven, hardworking, humble pool champion. I knew he would be the one person who could really understand me.

It happened inside an elevator after I lost a devastating tournament match that knocked me out of the event. I was furious, feeling down on myself for my poor play, and I was waiting for George to tell me everything was okay. But he didn't. George didn't try to explain away my defeat. He just walked out of that elevator into our hotel room, and he was silent.

I was the No. 1 pool player in the world and I had lost my match that night. Of course, losing is part of the package. When you compete, there are going to be losses, but some are more painful than others. I was devastated. I had played terribly and I was unfocused. I was embarrassed and disappointed.

But one thing I always made sure of, no matter how tough the defeat, was that I would be a gracious competitor. I would always stick around after my matches to make sure that every person who wanted an autograph from me or a photo with me would get it. I stood around after that match, faking a smile as I interacted with fans.

When all of that was over and George and I got in the elevator, there was dead silence for the first time. I turned my smile off, and I waited. I didn't want George to try to be nice about it. I was just waiting for him to say something stupid that pissed me off, like, "It's alright. You'll get them next time," or, "She got really lucky against you," or anything other than what he said.

Which was nothing.

George understood. He was a pool player, after all. He knew nothing he could say was going to make me feel any better. He understood I needed time to cool off.

As we got off the elevator and walked down the hall to our hotel room, I was still waiting for George to say something stupid, but he never did.

I walked in and plopped myself down on the bed and stared at the ceiling. I knew he would eventually have to say something comforting and I'd have to thank him, even though I really didn't want to talk about it at all. George didn't try to lay on the bed next to me. He just went over to the window, stood there, and looked outside. The room was filled with silence. It was wonderful. George let me have my silence.

When I was finished stewing, I said, "George, are you hungry? I'm hungry." He was hungry, too. As we headed out to eat, all I could think of in that moment was, "I am definitely marrying this man. He understands me. He gets me. He is my soulmate."

George quickly booked a flight to New York City to meet my parents, to ask for my hand in marriage, and I went with him. I tried to coach him beforehand on how to behave. "Let them do most of the talking." "Be respectful, and don't cross your arms, because that is a sign of disrespect."

It didn't matter how cool and wonderful George was with my parents. It wouldn't have mattered what he said. My mother and father, who both loved that George was a Christian, still thought it was too soon for us to get married. They thought we were rushing into this whole thing. They told us we needed to take our time.

In New York, George and I listened to what my parents had to say, and then I privately told them it was happening. We were going to get married, whether it was with their blessing in New York City or not.

If not, George and I were considering getting married in Hawaii, with just our friends and closest family who wanted to be there. I didn't want that. I desperately wanted my parents' blessing.

Eventually, my mom agreed to our marriage, but she wanted to plan the wedding and have it in New York in front of our family and friends. That was fine with me, because George and I were insanely busy traveling to be with each other at our tournaments. For all my mom had sacrificed for me, I agreed to do it her way.

Six months later, on January 6, 1996, I married George Breedlove at the Astoria World Manor in Queens, New York. The wedding inside that regal banquet hall was beautiful. The Astoria had majestic ballrooms, sparkling chandeliers, and huge dance floors.

George and I were so in love as we said our vows. It was absolutely magical.

But hours later, as the morning of January 7 dawned, the infamous Blizzard of 1996 slammed New York City. That storm lasted 37 hours, dropped an average of two inches of snow per hour, and it brought the city to a complete halt.

Residents were told to stay home, businesses were shut down, airports were shut down, the streets were shut down, and people were left stranded.

All my wedding guests at the Marriott were stranded, too. They couldn't go anywhere. The snow drifts had literally covered their cars. Food was limited, because trucks weren't bringing in deliveries. I felt so bad because George's parents and grandparents had traveled from Indiana, and my whole family was there, too. And we were all just stuck.

Lucky for George and I, we hadn't planned a traditional honeymoon. There was pool that had to be played. Days after our wedding, we were both supposed to be in Santa Rosa, California, for the ESPN World Open 9-Ball Championship, which featured the biggest prize money in pool at the time.

At first, it looked like we would have to miss the tournament, but somehow George managed to get a rental car out of New York.

We drove from New Jersey to Pennsylvania, which was also in a state of emergency. No cars were supposed to be on the road, but we drove on the highway anyway, very slowly, through ice and snow.

Then, all of a sudden, there was a wall of snow right in front of us. The highway, literally, just ended. We turned around to exit the highway, and started driving on side roads, when a police officer pulled us over.

That state trooper was ready to impound our car. No one was supposed to be out driving, he told us very sternly. But George started explaining the situation. "This is The Black Widow," he told the trooper. "We've got to get to her tournament. She is going to be on ESPN."

Somehow, George smoothly talked the trooper into letting us go, letting The Black Widow go. That trooper told us he was a fan, gave us directions on how to take the backroads, and wished us good luck.

After making it to the airport and then taking three different flights, I finally arrived in Santa Rosa, but I was in a bad way. We'd been traveling for two days without showers. We were exhausted and hungry.

It had been so stressful. We were always running to catch the next layover. The likelihood of us making it to our matches in time seemed nearly impossible. But I was amazed watching George in action, negotiating rental cars, driving through scary terrain on icy roads, keeping track of our bags, figuring out flights.

The whole time I just kept thinking, "This guy is amazing." George took charge and did whatever it took to get us there. I hadn't dated a ton of men before George, but none of them had his take-charge personality. With my type-A personality, I had learned quite early that if something needed to be done right, I had to do it myself. I always felt like I had to figure things out.

But with George, I was good. I could relax. I could loosen the reins, because he could handle it and get us there. And he did. He got us to our destination for that match.

Inside the bathroom of the airport, I dunked my head under water at the sink. I ran to the limo that was waiting to take us to the tournament, then changed my clothes and tried to towel dry my hair as we drove.

After we were dropped off, I walked very briskly to my match while attempting to pop my contact lenses into my eyes. I made it to the table with seven minutes to spare, seven minutes before my match would have been called a forfeit.

Somehow, after all of that, and after playing my heart out in that tournament, I won the whole thing, beating Allison Fisher 7–2 in the finals with a $68,500 payout for first place as the new Mrs. George Breedlove. It was absolutely insane.

I remember feeling so lucky to have George as my husband, this strong man who had miraculously gotten me to that tournament. This strong man, my new husband, who I knew was going to be there for me no matter what.

In the early years of our marriage, I always felt lucky to have George, who was very romantic. He always denied he was romantic, but he was. George was not a great singer, but he would sing a few country songs to me. He wrote down the lyrics to "I Think About It All the Time" by John Berry.

The way you laugh, the way you cry / The way that you smile without meaning to / The way you look me in the eye / I think about it all the time.

Next to each line, George wrote what I meant to him.

George would talk about how he remembered what I was wearing the first time he saw me: a simple black dress. He was so sweet, and he was so supportive of my pool game.

As newlyweds, we did everything together. George would go with me to my tournaments and I would go with him to his. Everything was great when we were living in L.A., playing pool and being parents to George's two daughters from his previous marriage, Olivia and Morgan.

I was always a very caring stepmother. I truly loved and adored Olivia and Morgan, who, to me, were my daughters that I shared with their biological mom. I loved George so much and those were his little girls. When we were living in L.A., we would fly to Indiana to see the girls where they lived, and we would fly them to L.A. to spend time with us.

I understood what a father meant to a little girl. I had always missed my biological father, John Tak, and I was always talking to George about that. And as I said, George was the one who, without telling me first, drove me to San Francisco to reunite with my biological father. And even though it was a wonderful reunion, it brought back memories and emotions I had tried to hide for 20 years.

As George and I were going to bed that night, I started pouring my heart out, trying to explain to him how much it hurt, and how much I missed not having my dad in my life growing up.

George was hearing all of my sorrow, for the first time, from a daughter's point of view, and he started thinking about his own daughters. He had just moved to L.A., away from his two little girls, and they were growing up without a dad.

I'll never forget that night in bed, as I looked over at George, I saw the tears in his eyes. I saw the tears rolling down his face.

"We need to move to Indiana, don't we?" I asked him.

"You would do that?" George asked me. He was in shock. I don't think he ever thought for one moment I would ever leave L.A., especially at the height of my pool career.

"Absolutely," I said to George. "As a daughter who grew up without her dad, absolutely. Let's do it."

I'm not sure George ever really grasped the sacrifice I made moving to the Midwest. I was the No. 1 women's pool player in the world, living minutes from Hollywood. I was in my prime and I had all the connections. I had every opportunity to go into movies and do auditions. I gave up a lot. But I never regretted it. I had my priorities straight. I knew family came first. Anyway, my priority was always to be the best player in the world, not the most famous. I thought I could do that just as well in Indiana as I could in L.A. After all, I married a professional; at the very least, I could play pool with him all the time.

When I made a cameo appearance in the 1999 Walt Disney movie, *The Other Sister,* I had no real reason to be in that movie. But the film's director, Garry Marshall, was a big fan of mine and he said he wanted me in his film.

Without a script, I flew out and met Garry, Juliette Lewis, Giovanni Ribisi, Diane Keaton, and Tom Skerritt. I remember being on that set and Garry telling me that I was a star. He brought me an ice cream pop and he signed a dollar bill.

"You should be very proud of yourself. This means you're a star," he said to me. "Keep this and remember that this is just the beginning."

I knew it wasn't. By the time Garry called me to do that movie, I had already packed up and moved to Indiana. I had made my choice.

When I initially married George, I pictured us living in L.A. as I continued to build my game, my name, and my brand. Instead, I decided that family, specifically George's daughters, should come before business, so we moved to Indiana.

> "We could have been doing all kinds of stuff had Jeanette lived in New York or L.A. In Indianapolis, those lucrative opportunities weren't one block away. Over the course of her career, moving to Indiana cost Jeanette hundreds of thousands of dollars."
>
> —Tom George, Lee's longtime manager

George may not have ever realized the sacrifice I made, but that doesn't matter. I didn't move to Indiana to get credit or be a martyr. I did it because I really felt like Olivia and Morgan needed their father. I thought it would be worth it. I thought our marriage would always be wonderful.

Two years into our marriage, we settled into a house in Carmel, in a very upper-class neighborhood George picked out. But we were still 40 minutes away from his daughters, who lived in Mooresville.

I remember wondering why we had moved thousands of miles across the country to be this far away from his daughters. George assured me Mooresville wasn't a town I could survive in. I'm still not sure what he meant by that.

Everything between George and I changed after we moved to Indiana. It was like the beginning of the end of our marriage, though our marriage lasted nearly 20 years. When we were living in L.A., George and I did everything together. In Indiana, George became more independent.

He was gone all the time working, and I was by myself a lot. George became an entrepreneur, trying his hand in all sorts of businesses—gazebos, fencing, decks, and construction. When we first got married, we agreed I'd pay the bills, and for the first time, he could just focus on pool. I made enough for both of us and I believed in him. He was ranked sixth on the men's Pro Billiards Tour, so he was nothing to sneeze at. But not long after that, the PBT folded. There were other fledgling men's tours that tried to make it but so many of the top guys were bumping heads, nothing ever grew. He was at the top of his game. I think it was really disheartening for him. On the other hand, the WPBA contract was exploding.

About a year into our marriage, while I continued to play, George set out to get his furniture business going again. Los Angeles was a totally different market than he was used to, so it was a challenge. However, it was not long after that when we had the meeting with my biological father, which resulted in George and I beginning to talk about him missing his girls, and the decision to move to Indiana.

George and I started drifting apart, little by little by little over two decades. We had separated twice and were heading toward divorce.

As I grew older, I realized that it was more important for our personalities to mesh than our hobbies. I learned that I really liked companionship and doing things together. George was very much an introvert.

Looking back, I honestly don't think George and I should have gotten married, but I was so sure he was the guy that I didn't listen to my friends and family who said it was too soon. Making a marriage work for a lifetime takes a lot of compromise and understanding. I thought that if two good people, two Christian people, loved each other, we could get through anything. But that was not the case.

When George and I agreed to move to Tampa, I was able to set the arrival date to be the day before I was contracted to do a trick-shot show for a grand opening of Tampa's beautifully designed Bass Pro Shops. I had underestimated how much time it would take to organize the transition and pack all our things in preparation for the move, because I didn't know that George was going to take a salmon fishing trip in Alaska for two weeks—the week before and during the week that we had originally planned the move to Tampa. I also wrongly assumed that, considering my recent ankylosing spondylitis diagnosis and having to manage all the girls while he was gone, he would help us pack, at the very least, some of the kids' things, even if he didn't help with anything else.

So as the moving day quickly approached, I started panicking. My friends Dianna, Marlene, and Marc and I ended up frantically throwing the rest of our things in boxes and bins, while caring neighbors stopped by to drop off any extra empty boxes for us to use to pack more of our things. We made sure we emptied and cleaned our house in Indy before my upcoming celebrity appearance at Bass Pro Shops' grand opening in Tampa so that we wouldn't have to come back twice. I already had a really tight travel schedule planned for the rest of the year, with tournaments in the U.S. and China, a European military tour, and several corporate appearances throughout the U.S. So I had to hit the ground running once I got to Tampa to ensure a smooth transition operating the business. I was very alone and very sad for a long time. I knew this marriage was ending after my surgery.

In 2015, nearly 20 years after George and I said those magical vows in the Astoria in Queens, New York, we divorced.

I don't regret my marriage to George Breedlove, although I would advise anyone not to rush into marriage. Being in love with someone isn't enough to make a lasting marriage. You have to be able to communicate through disagreements in a healthy manner and both be willing to compromise a lot. If you're the kind of person that just buries things, resentments build and an unhappy marriage becomes inevitable. Still, it was because of our marriage that my biggest, most wonderful dreams came true, the dreams that filled my heart and soul.

Because of my marriage to George, I became the mother to six incredible, amazing children.

CHAPTER 21

FROM DESPERATELY WANTING A BABY TO A GRATEFUL MOTHER OF SIX

LONG BEFORE I DREAMED OF BEING A BILLIARDS STAR, I dreamed of being a mother. I always knew I wanted to have a baby. But not just one baby. I always dreamed of having a big crew of little ones—five, six, maybe even seven children running around the house—who would grow into rambunctious teens and become amazing, successful adults who would make a difference in this world.

I always pictured a house full of love and laughter, with a big, beautiful family making incredible memories, decorating Christmas trees, going to pumpkin patches, and hunting for Easter eggs.

When I married George Breedlove in 1996, I became a 24-year-old stepmother, and I liked that. I loved Morgan and Olivia dearly, and they made me want to have a baby of my own even more.

In the early years of our marriage, George and I talked a lot about having children. I made it clear to him during those deep, intimate conversations we would have, how desperately I wanted to be a mother. But I was young, and I was on the cusp of a superstar pool career.

While I would have been happy to get pregnant right away, George and I knew we had plenty of time. At least we thought we did. We could travel the world together, competing, and enjoying being newlyweds. Then we could have children.

Plus, if George and I were going to have kids, he had a vasectomy that needed to be reversed.

George had gotten his vasectomy very, very young. By the time he was 20, George was married to his high school sweetheart and they had two daughters. He didn't want any more kids, not only because of financial reasons but because the relationship between him and his wife was often rocky, so George had a vasectomy.

But when he and I got together, George told me he loved kids, and he'd be thrilled to have more children, if that's what I wanted. We were in a much better position financially to raise kids than he had been before and that made him more comfortable with the idea. George reversed his vasectomy.

But even after that procedure, we couldn't get pregnant. We knew we were dealing with very few of George's soldiers, because we had been married 10 years, and nothing. I thought maybe there was something wrong with me, so I went to doctors, but they never found any medical reason I couldn't get pregnant.

I went to George and told him how scared I was. "It's not working. I don't think we're going to get pregnant naturally. We've got to do something."

We started injections, and took different medicines, but nothing worked. Finally, we tried in vitro fertilization. We spent $28,000 on a procedure that had a 14 percent chance of success. But that didn't work, the first or the second time. We even froze the extra embryos, but they didn't survive.

I can't put into words how painful that was, waiting every month in anticipation, only to be disappointed. Not just month after month after month, but year after year after year. I was giddy at the thought of getting pregnant, then every time my period came, it was devastating.

I desperately wished that I didn't want children, that I hadn't always dreamed of a big family. But I did want children, and I wanted a big family, and not getting that was pure torture.

Then one day, in an instant, all the torture disappeared when, in an ironic twist of fate, I became a mother to my first newborn daughter, Cheyenne. I still believe to this day that me becoming a mother was an outright miracle that began, where else? At a pool tournament in May 2004.

At that tournament, the Billiards Congress of America Open, a Bible study was being held for the players, and I wanted to go for spiritual nourishment. But to be completely honest, I almost didn't go, even though I really wanted to.

The Bible study began at 8:30 AM and I liked to sleep in at tournaments. I liked to wake up without an alarm so that I knew I was fully rested. Mornings are also tough for me because of pain from arthritis and scoliosis.

Can't we do this at noon? I remember lamenting to whomever would listen. God must have been listening.

For some reason, I woke up at 8:00 AM the morning of the Bible study, and I wasn't just awake. I was wide awake, and I was feeling really energetic. I remember being mad about that. I thought I needed more sleep. I had a tournament to play that night.

I forced myself to stay in bed, shoved my head underneath the pillows, and I tried to fall back asleep. But I couldn't fall back asleep.

"Okay, God," I thought to myself, as I begrudgingly dragged myself out of bed. "I hear you loud and clear."

I was already half an hour late to the Bible study by that time, but I threw on some clothes, quickly made myself presentable, and went downstairs to a conference room in the hotel. The pool players were already in the middle of their devotion.

I sat down, started listening to our preacher and friend, Roy Dodson, and I was moved. I was really inspired. I can't exactly explain it.

Each of us was asked to tell the group something we would like a prayer for. As they went around the circle, the requests were heart wrenching—relatives who had cancer, people who had lost their home in a fire, an uncle in the early stages of dementia, a grandfather who was on his deathbed.

When it was my turn to ask for prayer, the only thing on my mind was that I wanted a baby. I wanted to be a mom. I poured my heart out to those other players.

"I know that this seems really silly compared to all the other things you guys are praying for, but I really always thought that I would have a big family, and I want children," I told the group. "I just don't know what to do. Do I keep trying, or do I adopt?"

George and I had been married nearly 10 years, and I was 33 years old. We tried medicine, injections, and in-vitro, all with no success. And, by that time, I had endured two miscarriages. I had never been so sad, so deeply sad, and numb.

"It just doesn't seem like it's meant to be," I said near tears, as the room began to pray for me. "I feel hopeless a lot of the time. All I ever wanted was to be a mother."

When the Bible study was over, I walked toward the elevator, still feeling really moved and, in a way, refreshed. There is something about pouring out your heart and soul. It makes you vulnerable and, in my mind, I had given my worries to God.

As I got ready to get on the elevator to go back to my room, I heard a voice call out, "Jeanette." It was one of the men from the Bible study.

"I just wanted to tell you that I was very moved by your testimony," that man said to me. "As I was praying, I felt God speaking to me, wanting me to talk to you. You said you've tried to have a baby every way that you could. The one thing you haven't tried is adoption. Maybe God means for you to try something else. Maybe the floodgates will open, and you'll be blessed with a baby."

I'm not sure why that man's words resonated with me so strongly that morning, but for the first time in years, I felt an amazing peace with my situation, and I felt at peace with the idea of adopting. I went to George after that Bible study and I told him that we were going to adopt a baby.

George didn't flinch. He wholeheartedly agreed. We both knew, after all, that no matter how we had a baby, biologically or through adoption, we would love them as our own. We would shower them with affection and we would make them feel like the most wonderful children in the world.

We quickly started researching adoption agencies and found one that was perfect for us, Holt International, an agency that was both Korean and Christian. The very next day, I made the call to start the process of bringing a child into our lives. I was ecstatic. Maybe I would finally get to be a mom.

Two days later, a huge packet of papers arrived in the mail: forms that needed to be filled out, requests for medical and financial information, passports, and our views on faith. The forms were so detailed, asking for so much information, George and I worked hour upon hour the entire week to fill them out.

On Sunday, one week after I had gone to that Bible study, we spent all day finishing the papers to mail out on Monday. I breathed a sigh of relief, said a little prayer, and I headed off to the sweet 16 birthday party for my goddaughter, Gabby Seo. George said he was too mentally drained to go after dealing with so much paperwork.

I was tired too, but I couldn't miss that party.

Gabby and her family had been our neighbors when George and I first moved to Indiana from L.A. We lived in a Carmel neighborhood filled with White people but, in our cul-de-sac, right across the street from George and I, was one Korean family—Gabby, Jenny, their brother Danny, and their parents.

I would go over to their house whenever I was craving authentic Korean food. I knew I would not be disappointed. Their kitchen smelled like my apartment growing up: kimchi, bibimbap, miyeok guk, and bulgogi.

But usually the Seo kids were at our home. George and I were known as the family with the fun house in the neighborhood. We had all kinds of board games. We would bake cakes and play ball in the yard, and we had a heated, in-ground pool with a diving board.

Gabby, Jenny, and Danny would come over to our house a lot, almost every day, and so did just about every kid in the neighborhood. We loved all of them, and they loved us and our girls, Morgan and Olivia.

We would have contests in the pool to see who could make the biggest splash, the smallest splash, or concoct the most creative dive. One time, we set out to make the neighborhood's largest sundae. On our kitchen island I put out all kinds of flavors of ice creams, with different, fun, toppings—gummy bears, M&M's, sprinkles, whipped cream, and syrups.

Then each kid took their turn decorating their own ice cream pile on a huge silver platter. After covering the whole thing in whipped cream, we all dug in.

Those times with all those kids were some of the best years of my life. I was a stepmother, but I didn't have any children of my own, and I fell in love with the neighborhood kids, especially Gabby, Jenny, and Danny. They became like family to me.

When George and I moved from Carmel to Mooresville, we stayed in touch with Gabby's family, but we were 40 miles apart. We didn't get to see them much, not like we used to. It broke my heart to leave Carmel, to leave all those kids.

So, it was very important to me that I be there for Gabby's sweet 16 birthday party. I had no idea that party would change my life forever.

By the time I arrived at Gabby's party, it was raining, and the festivities had been moved inside. I walked over to the dining room table and sat down to catch my breath and dry off. Across the table was a man named Court. He was the Seos' youth pastor.

I introduced myself to Court, who already knew of me because the kids had talked about me, and explained why I had shown up late to Gabby's party. I told him George and I had been working on those adoption papers, pages and pages of forms, to prove we were worthy of having a baby of our own.

Before Court could respond, out of nowhere, I heard this little pipsqueak of a voice ring in my ears, "Did you say you're going to adopt?"

That voice belonged to Minyoung, a tiny, 17-year-old girl, who slid her chair back from the table to reveal a little bump on her stomach. "I was thinking about giving my baby up for adoption," she said to me.

Minyoung was one of Gabby's friends, and she was thin, frail, and very, very shy. I felt sorry for her, and, at the same time, I was elated at the thought of having a baby. I immediately told Minyoung, as we sat at the dining room table, that I would adopt her baby.

Looking back, I know that wasn't appropriate. It was rash. But Minyoung was thrilled. "Are you serious?" she asked me. Yes, yes, yes! I was serious.

Minyoung asked if George and I wanted to meet with her and the baby's father. Of course, we did. Two days later, we met Minyoung and her boyfriend at a grill that served burgers, chicken tenders, and onion rings. I was struck by how young and fragile they seemed. They were just a couple of teenagers, and they were under a lot of pressure.

Minyoung had desperately wanted to keep her baby. Court and the church started collecting donations and buying things for her that she'd need as a new mom. They tried to help her fill out forms to get financial assistance as a 17-year-old single mother.

But as time passed, it started to become clear that giving her baby up for adoption might be the best thing for Minyoung and for the baby. Without the support of her family, she wouldn't be able to manage on her own.

Minyoung was still in high school, after all, and her mother wanted her to give the baby up for adoption and never look back. If she kept the baby, her mother told Minyoung, she wasn't welcome back in the home. Her mom had been raised in a strict Korean household. Pregnant teens were considered shameful to the family.

It was a difficult time for Minyoung. She and her mother are on good terms now, but at the time, her mother was angry with her for getting pregnant. She wanted it to all go away. She wanted to pretend as if that baby never happened. I know that seems harsh, but I also know she wanted what was best for Minyoung's future, and this baby would change everything.

Two nights after our first meeting with Minyoung and the baby's father, George and I met with them again for dinner. We answered their questions, talked to them, and assured them we would take incredible care of their baby, giving that child unconditional love and security.

The next day, my phone rang and I heard the sweetest words I had ever heard. "We have decided we want you guys to be the parents of our baby," Minyoung said to me. She hadn't wanted to give her baby away blindly, to someone she didn't know.

She loved this baby and wanted to make sure that it was an open adoption so she could always see her daughter, so she could make sure her daughter knew that she wasn't thrown away or abandoned.

Instead, Minyoung loved her daughter so much she was willing to give her baby up for a better life than she could give her.

As I talked to Minyoung on the phone, I tried to stay calm, even though I was bursting inside. "This is amazing," I said to her. "Can you hold on one second?" I covered up the phone and I screamed in joy. I was finally going to have a baby.

When I calmed myself down, George and I got back on the line. I asked Minyoung when the baby was due. She was so tiny, I assumed she was five months along or, at most, six months. I was wrong.

The baby's estimated due date was Sunday, just days away, and just two weeks after that Bible study I had attended at the pool tournament, that Bible study where I prayed to become a mom. This was a miracle. I had no doubt in my mind about that.

But, Minyoung didn't have the baby that Sunday. I wasn't there for the birth, and that has always been one of my biggest regrets. I had a pro event to play in Peoria, Illinois, which seemed perfect, just three hours from my house. It wasn't in California, Atlanta, Chicago, or New York, the places I often traveled to for tournaments.

I figured I would go to Peoria and I would have plenty of time to get back if Minyoung went into labor. But while I was at the tournament, on June 11, 2004, Cheyenne was born. I wish I had skipped that tournament. I hate that I was more worried about getting points for my tour ranking. I hate what I missed.

I never thought about how many years I imagined myself in the hospital, looking in that room where they held the newborn babies. I missed all of the hospital experience with Cheyenne.

When I got the call that Cheyenne had been born, I wanted to get to the hospital as quickly as I could. But George called my friends Don Wardell, Stu Mattana, and my coach Bob Carman, and asked them to stall me from coming home. He wanted to surprise me. They were the ones who drove me, so I was dependent on them. They kept making excuse after excuse about why we couldn't leave. Finally, we piled into the car and they gave me a ride from Illinois to meet my baby daughter.

I wanted them to drive me straight to the hospital, but George told me I had to come home first. I didn't want to, but George was adamant. As soon as I arrived at our house, George covered my eyes and said he had a surprise for me. He had gotten me a gift for the birth of our baby.

I have to admit, I was a bit annoyed, and I was very impatient. It was sweet of George, but I just wanted to get to the hospital and see my daughter's face. I just wanted to hold her. Why couldn't he understand that?

I pleaded with George to give me the gift later. Instead, he positioned me on the couch, then he told me to open my eyes. When I did, standing in front of me was my stepdaughter, Olivia, holding Cheyenne. She laid my daughter in my arms.

George had planned all of this. He had told the guys to stall from driving me home from the tournament, because he wanted me to be in the privacy of our home, holding Cheyenne in my arms, three weeks to the day after I went to the Bible study and made the decision to adopt.

As I stared at my baby, this perfect person without a blemish on her skin, I was overwhelmed. I started bawling. George cried, too, as he watched me holding Cheyenne, our miracle.

I finally had what I wanted, my very own baby. I prayed so hard for 10 years for God to bless me with a baby. Here I was, three weeks later with a baby in my arms. I thought of that man who suggested adoption. He said, either you'll wait a long time because it's just not meant to be, or He means for you to adopt and the floodgates will open. I would call this the floodgates opening. Not only was a perfectly healthy, beautiful, half-Korean, half-Caucasian baby in my arms three weeks to the day that we prayed for me to have a baby, we also found out that since Minyoung was 17, she was still fully covered under her mother's health insurance. We didn't have a dime in medical expenses. We received tons of baby gear from what the church collected for Minyoung.

Here's the final kicker that made it clear to me that she was Heaven sent: it turned out that Court, the youth pastor who I met at Gabby's sweet 16, was only a youth pastor on the weekends. During the week, he was a family attorney, specializing in adoptions. Because he loved Minyoung and thought our plan to adopt her baby was a good idea, he offered to do the entire legal adoption for free. The only thing we ended up paying for was a $250 filling fee to the state for the mandatory home study. There is no doubt in my mind that God meant for me to adopt Cheyenne. We were so happy and so blessed.

As the weeks and months passed, I was enamored with Cheyenne. I was obsessed with being the best mother I could be. I took Cheyenne with me everywhere I went, to the grocery store, to the park, to the bank, and she traveled with me all over the world for my tournaments, including Austria, Taiwan, Japan, and China.

George thought it was a waste of money to travel with Cheyenne and a nanny. "Wouldn't it be easier and save us money if she just stayed home?" he would ask me. I promptly told George I hadn't waited this long to have a baby just to let someone else raise her. Either Cheyenne goes with me or both of us would stay home, and I'd stop working. Enough said. George never complained again.

I absolutely loved being a mother, and I was sure there was no way in the world I could ever love another human as much as I loved Cheyenne.

But that quickly changed in an incredible way when God blessed me with three more little—and not so little—humans to love and call my very own.

About a year and a half after Cheyenne was born, my son John Kang and his brother Billy came into my life, another miracle.

My cousin Esther, who grew up in that Brooklyn apartment building with me and was, and still is, more like a sister than a cousin, was married to Jin Han, a criminal defense lawyer in New York City. He happened to be representing a couple who had three sons.

When the couple was sent to prison, Esther and her husband started fostering the two younger boys, Billy and John, when they were 14 and 11 years old. They fostered them for three years, along the way having children of their own.

I thought it was incredible of Esther and her husband, considering they had babies and toddlers, but they didn't want to break up Billy and John. One summer, George and I had the boys stay with us to give Esther a break.

We fell in love with them, but they were a bit rough around the edges. They fought a lot, not just verbally but physically, too. At Esther's house, their fights caused holes in the wall and put dents in the refrigerator. I remembered being worried for her.

Not long after Billy and John stayed with us, Esther and her husband asked George and I to take a vacation with them over Christmas vacation. We rented a five-bedroom condo in Naples. On the last night, out of the blue, Esther and her husband sat George and I down.

By this time Billy was 17 and John was 14. Esther told us she was really worried about them and she needed to find a home for them. They had been through enough. The Han's home was not a permanent solution because they really didn't have any bedrooms for them.

In addition, they were going to a school where gun detectors and video monitors were the norm, due to the violence. They were living in a place where, if they didn't join a gang, they would not be safe. And if they did join a gang, they definitely would not be safe.

Esther and her husband didn't want to see Billy and John go into the foster care system and get split up. They didn't want to see their lives go down the wrong path. But they had several young children, a small apartment, and they could not give them the devotion they needed.

Sitting together that last night in Naples, Esther asked George and I to adopt the boys.

I remember telling her that she was crazy. There was no way. I was traveling around the world for tournaments, I was at the peak of my career, I had Cheyenne—I couldn't take on two teenage boys.

"These boys need a full-time mom, and I can't be that. I've got too much going on," I said. George and I told Esther we couldn't adopt them. But she didn't give up.

"Jeanette, your part-time is going to be way better than anyone else's full-time," she said. "You're going to give 100 percent. You're going to love them like your own."

George and I talked about it, we prayed about it, and we decided we couldn't leave Billy and John in the lurch. They couldn't be split up. In January 2006, we brought them to live with us in Mooresville, Indiana.

Because Billy was 17, set to graduate from high school in the spring and getting ready to start his freshman year at Syracuse University, we didn't adopt him legally. But he lived with us until that fall, and we became his loving godparents, with the blessing of his parents.

As Billy headed off to college, we bought his laptop, clothes, nice shoes, and anything he needed for his dorm. We set up a water delivery system to his room and we filled his cabinets with Ramen noodles. I would send Billy snack packs, Korean junk food, and I made sure John and I visited him in college, just to make sure he felt loved and welcomed. I wanted him to know that he had a home base, and that he had two people who were always there for him.

Because John was only 14, George and I knew he needed more than just a place to live, so we legally adopted him. I know it must have been so hard for his parents to sign over custody, but they had to so we could enroll John in high school.

He had been failing school in New York City, not attending class, and not trying. His family had been tossed upside down, and his parents were in prison. John didn't care about school, and who could really blame him?

George and I had to make him care about school, about his future, and that was tough. John always said I nagged at him. But that nagging, he knew, meant I loved him. I believed in him. I knew he could do much better than he was doing. I wanted him to know it. The only way he'd find that out is if I pushed him past his comfort zone. That's how he would find out how smart and capable he really was. Someone had to teach him to work hard in school. He needed that confidence. I told him, "John, I want you to know, you don't have to go to college to be happy or successful. College doesn't guarantee you a good future. It only gives you more opportunities. But if you don't learn to work hard, if you won't put your best effort in, then you'll just be wasting your time and money. If you think you'll be happy living frugally, working in a convenience store, then I will support you. But you have to decide right now, your freshman year, if you want to go to college. Because at this rate, with your grades and your reading level, there's no way you'll make it into any college." Heck, a couple teachers told me they didn't think he'd finish high school.

John didn't skip a beat. He said, quietly but confidently, "Don't worry. I'm going to college. That's for sure."

I said, "Okay then, John, if you're sure, then you've got a ton of work ahead of you. I know you can do it, I believe in you and I'm here for you. I'll support you in every way that I can, but you're going to have to do the work. Work harder than you ever have before." And by God, that's what he did. I hired tutors and study partners, we printed flash cards and bought books to study. I was so proud of him. He gives me a lot of credit for helping him, but really he deserves *all* the credit. He worked so hard because he knew that he wanted a bright future.

John joined the wrestling team at Mooresville High School and he worked his way up to varsity. He even coached fifth grade boys wrestling. He loved to play basketball. He loved to play with his little sister, Cheyenne. As he grew older, John said coming to Indiana to live with us was a turning point in his life.

Years later, John got a black widow spider tattoo on his left arm so he could always be reminded of where his life had been, and where he ended up.

> "My biological family went through some hard times. I wasn't necessarily making the best decisions. Jeanette stepped in, and the rest is history."
>
> —John Kang, Lee's son

By 2008, I had Cheyenne, who was four; John, who was nearly an adult; and my two stepdaughters, but I still longed for more children, more babies. After all, Cheyenne was a perfect baby. Why wouldn't I want more of that? George always wanted to make me happy. He didn't really want more kids, but he agreed to it. He said, "Okay, but just one more, that's it." I said that was fine. I was 38 at that point. Between now supporting four children—soon to be five—still suffering from so much pain, having to have uninsured surgeries because no insurance company wanted to cover a woman with my health history, and dwindling income because I was playing less and hurting more, I didn't think it would be wise to try to have more. Especially because George and I hadn't been happy together in years. We still loved each other, but we were growing apart. I didn't care though. I wanted to have another child whether we stayed together or not. We considered adopting again when a woman offered to be a surrogate. We hadn't even considered that. It turned out that she was not a good candidate, but it really got me thinking. In vitro didn't work for me, but maybe it would for a womb in another woman.

One day, I decided to put a post on a surrogacy website. I poured my heart out again. I kept it anonymous, posting about my and George's struggle becoming parents. I wrote about Cheyenne and

John, and I wrote how I still had a void in my heart. I wanted more children.

A woman named Angie, who lived in Indianapolis, was moved by my post, and she immediately called me. George and I met with Angie and her husband multiple times. We finally decided this felt right, very right.

Angie had a great job, she had two kids, and she loved being pregnant. She and her husband didn't want more children of their own, but Angie thought it would be a beautiful gift to give to someone, to give to me, to give me the gift of another child.

Through in vitro fertilization, doctors created embryos by fertilizing my eggs with George's sperm, and they implanted the embryos inside Angie. We were so excited when we found out she was pregnant with twins.

I was over the moon and immediately started ordering twin books, twin clothes, double strollers, and twin rockers. I started reading all the same baby books as I did with Cheyenne. I was nervous because of our previous miscarriages, but after the first trimester I let out a little sigh of relief.

We passed that mark and went to the 16-week ultrasound, where I was anxious to find out the genders of the babies. There we were with Angie lying on the table next to me. As the tech moved the ultrasound wand on Angie's stomach, she found the first twin, with a heart beating strong. I felt like crying. It was very emotional for me.

But then the tech moved the wand over to find the next baby. As she moved the scope around, we waited and waited and waited until finally she stopped on a very small, shriveled-up fetus. There was dead silence in that room. She didn't want to say it, and I didn't want to hear it. The second baby had died.

It's hard to describe going from feeling blessed, feeling like God blessed you with two babies after all the suffering and waiting, to losing one of those babies. I can tell you that the pain starts very deep in your gut, and it starts to eat at you from the inside out until it's all you think about.

It surprised me how deeply I could miss a child that was never born. For me, it was a complete loss, and that pain has never gone away. I can't help but think about this child that wasn't meant to be. I believed, from my past experiences, that everything happens for a reason, and that God has a greater plan. Have faith in Him and stay steadfast. But this time, like so many times before, it was hard to understand why things were happening in the moment. I became deeply depressed. But Angie was still carrying our daughter, Chloe, who was growing healthy and strong inside her womb. I tried to be happy, excited about Chloe, but the dark cloud remained. Still, I was very thankful. I prayed to God and thanked him for the healthy baby girl that I received from this angel, Angie.

Angie carried our biological baby for nine months. It was nothing short of an amazing, selfless act from a wonderful human being.

In October 2009, Chloe was born, a perfect and healthy, seven-pound, beautiful baby, our first—and probably last—biological child. I look back on that time, and I have only three words: *What a gift.* What a gift Angie had given to us.

We hired a photographer to take family photos, pictures of our family of seven. I could hardly believe it, but I now had five children—Morgan, Olivia, Cheyenne, John, and Chloe. In one photo, a tiny Chloe laid with pool balls all around her, with a pink, silk blanket on top of her, stitched with the words "Baby Widow," the same baby blanket that Cheyenne had as a newborn. I wasn't sure my life could get any better.

Then, eight weeks after Chloe was born, I walked into the bathroom with a pregnancy test in my hand, and my world was turned upside down. Never, in a million years, had I seen this coming.

My body had been feeling different, so I decided to rule out pregnancy. I will never forget going to the bathroom to take the test and seeing the positive result. I could not believe it, so I took another test and then another test. It didn't matter how many times I tried. They were all positive.

I started bawling. My personal assistant at the time, Dianna, who eventually became one of my closest, most loyal and dear friends, heard me crying in the bathroom, knocked on the door, and asked me what was wrong.

I couldn't get myself up from the toilet to utter anything that made sense because, honestly, nothing made sense. Finally, I got the strength to unlock the bathroom door and hand my positive pregnancy test to Dianna. I stood looking at her with tears running down my face, my black makeup and eyeliner all smeared.

Dianna told me she couldn't understand why I was crying. I tried to explain it to her. Why, at one of the happiest times of my life with my new daughter, Chloe, would I have to endure another miscarriage? I was sure there was no way I would actually carry this baby full term. I never had before—and now I was 39 years old.

I knew for the next couple of months I would be tortured as a tiny human grew inside of me, only to be devastated as the baby was ripped away. And those months that followed became one of the most painful and torturous times for me and also one of my biggest regrets—I didn't let myself enjoy the one natural pregnancy I had.

I tried to be happy but George and I hadn't been really happy as a married couple for at least 10 years. I became withdrawn. I was scared.

From the age of 13 on, I had endured countless surgeries to strengthen my back. Because of my severe scoliosis, doctors thought I might never be able to carry my own child, but as usual I defied the odds in too many ways to count.

Eleven months after Chloe was born, I gave birth to my third daughter, Savannah.

> "Before she delivered our daughter, she was going to get an epidural, only they couldn't find her spine. Three inches of scar tissue had formed from all her back surgeries. After two hours, and 100 pokes of the needle, they stopped trying. She delivered the baby naturally."
>
> —George Breedlove,
> Jeanette's then-husband, *ESPN The Magazine*

The ability to carry my own child, and to give birth to my own child, was an amazing experience, an indescribable experience. It was something I had always dreamed of, and it became something I was sure would never happen.

Yet, somehow, by the grace of God, with a lot of prayers, too many angels around me to name, and a few miracles, I went from desperately wanting a baby to being the mother of six. I did it in the most untraditional of ways, as a stepparent, by adoption, by surrogacy, and by natural birth.

And those six children are, far and away, the greatest accomplishments of my life—even greater than the gold medal that meant my own parents finally, once and for all, accepted me.

CHAPTER 22

A GOLD MEDAL AND SWEET VINDICATION

MY PARENTS WERE SHARING MY SUCCESS with everyone in the family, telling all their friends, and talking about me to strangers. That felt absolutely wonderful to me. Finally, my parents were proud of me. Finally.

It was 1994 and I was the No. 1 women's pool player in the world. I had proven to my parents that billiards wasn't some silly little obsession. It wasn't some convoluted, far-flung dream. I was only 23 years old, and I had skyrocketed to the No. 1 ranking in a very short time.

I was being called an outright pool phenomenon, and I was becoming a media sensation.

Finally, after all the late nights my parents worried about me as I was out playing billiards, after all of the arguing, after all the pastors and family members praying for me at every church gathering, my parents were actually proud of me.

They were genuinely proud of me for making it big in billiards.

Still, my dad would tease me, though he said the words in a pretty serious voice. "Jeanette, you know I'm proud of you, but when are you going to be in the Olympics?"

Of course, I wanted to go to the Olympics. Every elite athlete dreams of winning an Olympic gold medal. Unfortunately, for me, pocket billiards wasn't recognized as an Olympic sport at the time.

I would try to explain that to my dad, but it didn't stop him from asking me, the next time he saw me, when billiards would be in the Olympics.

The billiards community was vehemently fighting to make billiards an Olympic sport and, in 1996, they decided to bring me into their Olympic fight as the top American player. I was chosen to travel with the executive director of the Billiard Congress of America, Stephen Ducoff, to stand before the International Olympic Committee. We were there to try to convince the committee that pool was a sport that should be on its roster.

I was honored and very excited to explain what makes billiards just like any other ball sport. You can't just know the right moves, like in chess. You have to have the stroke, the knowledge, the accuracy, the lucidity, the consistency, and the heart to excel at this beautiful game. My passion came through as they asked me questions. They smiled and nodded. They seemed thoroughly interested in pocket billiards.

For the next two years, the board members of the Billiard Congress of America, and the newly formed World Confederation of Billiards Sports (WCBS), worked with the International Olympic Committee, continuing its fight.

In 1998, their hard fought battle was won when pool was officially designated an Olympic sport. I was thrilled. I remember being so incredibly happy when I got that phone call. The only way I can describe it is that it felt like I might finally be considered a true athlete. An official athlete.

Except, it wasn't really official, at least not in my mind. Pool may have been dubbed an Olympic sport, but billiards players from across the world would not be competing in the summer or in the winter games.

If pool was ever to be part of those games, the Olympic committee said, it would probably be as an exhibition sport, not for players to compete for a medal. I knew that was part of the normal Olympic committee process, to eventually raise the sport to the echelon of competing for a medal, but it seemed doubtful to happen anytime soon. Maybe we were just paving the way. It was so disappointing.

It was sad. It seemed pretty certain that I would never be an Olympic gold medalist, standing at the podium as the national anthem played and the American flag was flown, representing my country as one of their sports heroes. I was so disappointed.

But in 2001, I got a very important call. I would be representing the United States in the World Games in Akita, Japan, as pool made its debut as a sport.

In the sport of pool, the equivalent to earning a gold medal at the Olympics is winning a gold medal at the World Games, an 11-day, international contest, much like the Olympics, typically taking place every four years (the year following the summer Olympics), featuring sports that are not part of the Olympic Games.

The World Games definitely wasn't anything to sneeze at. I was absolutely ecstatic and grateful. I was also really worried.

That call couldn't have come at a worse time. I might have been the top-ranked American woman at that time, but I was lying in bed, recovering from three back-to-back surgeries—the first one for my neck, the second surgery for my back, and the third one for my shoulder.

By that time, I was 30 years old, and I had herniated a disc in my neck that made playing pool impossible. I literally could not bend down and tilt my head up to see anything on the billiard table. I was in so much pain that all I wanted to do was lie in bed with the lights turned off, wallowing in the darkness.

When doctors told me I would have to undergo neck surgery to keep playing pool, I decided I might as well take care of my other issues, my shoulder and my back. I had bursitis and bicep tendonitis in my left shoulder. And, of course, my back was always giving me trouble due to my pseudarthrosis, which developed due to the spinal fusion I had for my severe scoliosis not healing properly.

By 2001, I'd been suffering from severe back pain for 30 years. After swearing to myself that I'd never go through back surgery again, all I could do was push through the pain, but year after year, it only got worse. The years of bending over with a fused spine, pseudarthrosis, and bulging discs, was catching up with me. I'd also been suffering from bursitis and bicep tendinitis for about 15 years. I just kept playing with that bad shoulder as I was grinding bone on bone. But after I injured my neck—resting for two months, taking time off the tour, hoping it would get better—I was forced to give up my previous conviction about surgery. By the time I finally went to my orthopedic doctor, Terry Trammell, took all the appropriate tests, made a plan, and scheduled the surgery, eight months had passed. It just took a while for me to accept that I had to stop competing. I was so worried that if I stopped I would lose my ranking and fans would forget about me. I had worked too hard for my skills, my ranking, and my brand to just let it all slip away. What if I never got my game back? I'd never taken even a week off of pool up until that point.

After enduring those three, strenuous surgeries, one right after the other, I wore a big neck brace, a back brace, and a sling for my left shoulder. I would hobble in all those gadgets using a walker around the cul-de-sac in my Indiana neighborhood, where my then-husband, George Breedlove, and I lived.

I'm sure I looked pretty pitiful to the neighbors who looked out their windows and saw me shuffling around.

One day, after hobbling around the neighborhood, I went back to my house, ready to relax in a recliner, when the phone rang. That was the call when I learned that, finally, I was going to get to compete for a medal for the first time in billiards history.

There was just one problem, a major problem. The World Games were set to begin August 22, and that was just weeks away. I had less than two months, a terrifyingly short amount of time, to prepare to win a medal. I hadn't been playing pool for eight months. I'd lost all confidence in my game. After that phone call, I started practicing again, but I was playing awful. I didn't know what to do.

When I was living in L.A., I pounded the table, playing every single day, every minute I could. When George and I moved to Indiana to be with his two daughters, I didn't practice as much. I didn't know anyone in Indianapolis. And George, who was now in his hometown with his friends and his family, was in his element. The men's tour had fallen apart and George decided to focus all his energy on growing his outdoor patio furniture business and worked from early in the morning until well past dinner. The man I married that used to play pool with me every day was gone. I was alone so much. I bought a brand new Diamond table, which were the best tables on the planet as far as most pros were concerned.

Still, playing by myself was boring, and little by little, I started playing less pool. I was attached to the kids, and all the other kids in the neighborhood. I loved spending time doing everything and anything with them, and when George had any free time, he joined in the fun. Our house was the fun house. I eventually made a few more friends that I could practice with, but it wasn't every day like it was in L.A. I was having fun with the neighborhood kids and their parents loved us. For the first time, I felt like I fit in. I belonged in that neighborhood and I was so happy. Happy in a way that I hadn't experienced ever before. Happy in ways that had nothing to do with pool.

There were so many distractions. I still worked every morning for five to six hours a day, making phone calls, doing interviews, and booking appearances. I'd hired a personal assistant to help with managing my busy travel schedule, booking flights, doctors appointments, bookkeeping, updating my website, etc. I was making great money. But there weren't a lot of tournaments around—there wasn't much competition—and my competitive spirit dwindled.

Luckily, I met a man named Bob Carman, who became my billiard coach and companion. George was always away working, and Bob was my companion. He had a camper set up on our property where he lived, and Bob was at my house every single day.

We would go into the pool room and practice. Bob would set up shots, we would work out our strokes, and Bob would try to keep me motivated. He saw how I was struggling with my game and he saw me in a total panic when I got the call to go to the World Games.

I had been waiting my entire career for this opportunity, to win a gold medal for my country. That was a huge deal to me, mostly because I knew it was something that would make my parents very proud. But I was definitely not on top of my game at that time, and I was so worried I would show up to Japan and disappoint not only my country, but my parents, too.

Bob quickly came up with an idea. He wanted to take me to see Jerry Briesath, a former pro who was a guru at teaching the stroking techniques of billiards. Jerry owned The Green Room in Green Bay, Wisconsin. It would be over a six-hour drive. With childhood arthritis and not being fully recovered from the surgeries, the idea was ridiculous—taking a long journey sitting in a car with a guy who, to me at the time, was just some old guy who was never a great champion. I thought, "Why waste four precious days making that journey." I wanted to stay home and do drills and maybe gamble a little to get some of my competitive toughness back. I remember asking Bob what this Jerry guy could teach me that I didn't already know. I had, after all, already risen to the ranking of the No. 1 women's player in the world.

Bob assured me that Jerry could teach me a lot.

I reluctantly agreed to meet with Jerry, on one condition: he was not allowed to try to change my stroke. Bob drove me to Wisconsin and, on that very first day, Jerry completely ignored my rule and started messing with my stroke.

Jerry asked me to shoot all sorts of shots at different speeds, from easy shots to extremely difficult shots, and, when I was finished, he brought me over to a monitor to watch what I had just done.

Until Jerry, I had never met a single person who ever talked about the mechanics of the stroke, the actual stroke itself. It was always about bank shots, how to kick at shots, how to cut the ball in, and what kind of sidespin to apply to the cue ball. I had never been taught about lining up your body, about clearance, about focus, and techniques such as the pendulum stroke and timing.

Jerry had been recording me as I was shooting those shots, which I didn't know at the time, and he had the camera focused, not on the table, or on the ball, but only on my bridge hand and arm.

I watched the video, aghast, as I would drop my elbow, instead of following through. I saw that I wasn't fully committed to the shot, which made me jump up on some strokes, or clench when I was trying to hit the ball hard. Jerry told me I should have a loose grip all the way through my swing, letting the timing and the speed accelerate through the follow through.

My mind was blown. I looked at the recording Jerry had made, I listened to what he told me, and I was disgusted with myself. *How did I get to No. 1 being undisciplined?*

I went back home and I practiced my new stroke, what Jerry had taught me in those few short days with him, and then I took that to the World Games in Japan. And what he taught me, I know now, helped me immensely. It took away a lot of my unforced errors. Jerry changed my stroke and he changed my game.

But I didn't know any of that as I headed into the World Games. I still didn't feel confident; I didn't feel dominant. I went in to compete for a gold medal for my country feeling completely unprepared. I hadn't been practicing even a tenth of the hours that my opponents had been practicing, and I was concerned.

I remember asking my mom to travel to Akita for the World Games with me, to be there to support me. She said she had to work.

> "I felt so bad that I didn't go with her because she invited me, she encouraged me to go with her, and I really missed that opportunity."
>
> —Sonja Lee, Jeanette's mother

In my first match, I struggled to win against a player who should have been easy for me. I honestly think that I was struggling more with jet lag than with my game. Due to the time difference, I was playing my 3:00 PM match in Japan when it was 3:00 AM in the United States. I was so fatigued. I just needed sleep.

After I pulled out a victory in the first match, as George and I left for our hotel, we walked past all these cute little shops, bars, pubs, and restaurants. As we went past one pub, its owner was out on the sidewalk, and he invited us in, luring us in with free hot sake. I loved hot sake.

I turned to George and said, "I could use a drink. Maybe that will help me go to sleep."

I didn't just have one drink that night. I was pretty well known in Japan, and the owner of that pub wanted to indulge me with all the hot sake I could ever want.

He brought an entire bottle of sake to our table, not just one glass, and then he brought another bottle, and then another (though the bottles weren't that big). Most of that night, it was just George and I drinking, plus a friend or two who saw us in the pub, and came in to drink with us.

That night after I won my first match at the World Games, I got kind of toasted on the sake, but I went back to the hotel room and I slept like a rock.

I woke up the next morning feeling so much better. George and I decided then and there what we had to do. Every single night of the World Games, we stopped by that pub, drank hot sake, and I slept like a baby.

I remember chuckling inside when people would ask me how I managed the jet lag. I never said a word. I never told them that my secret was hot sake. I went through the whole tournament feeling totally rested and on top of my game.

All these years later, I wish I had gone back to that pub and thanked the owner for how he, unknowingly, helped me. I guess this is me thanking him now.

I won the gold medal at the World Games in Akita, Japan, maybe because of the sake, and maybe because of Jerry and Bob, and maybe because I was desperate to show my parents I was the real deal.

No matter the reason, that was the most unforgettable moment of my career.

I won the gold medal against Karen Corr, the No. 1 player in the world at that time, who was known on the circuit as The Irish Invader. I literally trounced her. I thumped her, and it was awesome.

> "Karen Corr had come on the scene, and she became a rival. She was Joe Frazier to the Muhammad Alis of women's pool, players like Allison Fisher and Jeanette Lee. But Jeanette won the gold medal, which was a huge achievement. It is still the only time an American has won a gold medal."
>
> —Mike Panozzo, publisher of *Billiards Digest*

When I made the final shot against Corr that made me the World Games gold medalist in women's pool, I was ecstatic. I was so proud, so unbelievably happy, and I was on top of the world.

But, for some reason, I didn't feel teary-eyed, and I was positive that I would not cry the next day when I stood up at the podium to be presented with my gold medal.

Throughout the games I had watched the ceremonies for other sports, and I had watched as the medalists stood on stage as their country's anthems were played. It seemed like every single one of those athletes cried.

When it was my turn, I stood up on the giant outdoor stage the day after winning the final match, and there was a sea of athletes as far as I could see. They were all wearing different warmups with their country's colors and their country's flags.

It was a moment that I will never ever forget.

Standing on that podium with the American flag, I felt a breeze blowing on my face and I heard the roar of the crowd, all these elite athletes standing in front of me, chattering. But when the United States national anthem began to play, the entire crowd went silent.

As they raised the American flag and the anthem began to play, I started crying uncontrollably. I couldn't stop crying.

Everything hit me all in one moment—the patriotism, the pride, the magic of winning a gold medal. I felt the enormity of what I had done. My heart felt like it was in my throat. I couldn't breathe. I was trembling.

I had just represented my country, and everyone was standing in silence, recognizing the United States, because of me. Because of Jeanette Lee. It was an indescribable feeling. This was what it was all about.

When I got back to my hotel room in Japan, I made a phone call to New York City. I couldn't wait to make that phone call to my parents, and especially to my dad. He was the first person I thought of after I won the gold medal.

My mom answered the call. "Can you put dad on the phone?" I asked her. I could not wait to tell my dad what I had just done.

"Dad, I won the gold," I told him on that phone call. "I won the gold medal at the World Games."

"Oh, finally, finally, finally," he said to me. "Good, good. Good job, Jeanette."

It was a sweet vindication for me. It was absolutely amazing. Because, in that moment, I was sure that my parents, finally, were proud of me.

Not long after that, I did something I'm sure my parents would not be proud of. But until now, they've never heard this story. Very, very few people have heard this story—the tale of the only hustle of my life.

CHAPTER 23

THE ONLY HUSTLE OF MY LIFE?

IT WAS A HOT SUMMER DAY IN 2005 when I walked into the Indianapolis pool hall Claude & Annie's with a premeditated, dirty little scheme dancing in my head.

I laughed as I stuffed the back of my underwear with pads to create a bubble butt like J-Lo. I put on a clay prosthetic to widen my nose. I crammed my long black hair into a short, brown-and-red ombre wig. I put on cat-eye sunglasses.

I walked up to a pool table and I hustled some poor, unknowing player out of $700.

I only did it because of Rick Reilly, a popular, powerful writer with *Sports Illustrated.*

I had bumped into Reilly at the Super Bowl in February 2004 at Reliant Stadium in Houston, Texas. I was always going to Super Bowls, making corporate appearances, and walking Radio Row for interviews.

Radio Row is a phenomenon during Super Bowl week that includes more than 100 media outlets stationed in one giant ballroom, where

NFL stars, former players, and celebrities walk by doing impromptu interviews.

Reilly left his station, came up to me, shook my hand, and told me that he was a huge fan of mine. We stood there on Radio Row, talking about pool and about life, and we kind of hit it off. We exchanged phone numbers, and Reilly and I stayed in touch.

The following year, I ran into Reilly again at the Super Bowl at Alltel Stadium in Jacksonville, Florida. But this time, Reilly wasn't just there to shake my hand, tell me he was a fan, and do the small-talk thing. He was there to tell me he had an idea for me, an idea he called "sinister."

"Let me ask you something," Reilly said. "Do you think you could hustle someone?"

Reilly had an idea for his column in *Sports Illustrated*. He wanted to walk into a pool hall with me, the most famous women's player in the world, and hustle some poor sap out of hundreds of dollars without that guy knowing he was playing against The Black Widow. The article would be titled, "Doing the Hustle."

I told him I could, but it wouldn't work. I couldn't go into any billiard room in America, Europe, China, Taiwan, or the Philippines and not be recognized. Plus, I just don't get much joy out of stealing a guy's money by lying—cheating, as far as I was concerned. I also wasn't sure it was good for the image of pool. However, my husband at the time, George Breedlove, was all in on the idea. Publicity. Fame. A prominent *Sports Illustrated* columnist writing a story about me. He insisted that I could not let this opportunity pass me by.

Well, there were a few problems. One, I hated hustling. It was not my thing. I had been around it my entire career and I despised it.

In the world of pool, hustling was a regular thing, an every day, every minute, every second occurrence in billiards clubs throughout the United States. Players would use all sorts of tactics to disguise their skills, to lure an opponent of lesser skill into gambling at high stakes.

> "Pool hustling is a way of life that is frowned upon by society, but, if done correctly, it can become a very lucrative living...pool hustlers can generate anywhere from tens of thousands to even millions of dollars in a matter of a week. It all depends on who you play, when you play, and what halls you are able to conquer. Of course, these statistics aren't 100 percent accurate, due to the nature of the industry. They are just estimates that mostly depend on how smarmy the hustler is."
>
> —*The Standard Times*,
> "The Demonic Ways of a Pool Hustler," 2005

Smarmy is a perfect word for hustling. I have watched too many underhanded, deceitful, hustling matches to count over the years. I have watched arrogant, highly skilled men turn into bumbling idiots at the table, just to fake out their opponents.

In my mind, that was what pool hustling meant: fake antics and covert schemes. The hustlers would start by playing a few games, wagering small amounts or not betting at all. That created the perception that they were easy to beat, because they weren't confident enough to bet big money.

Some of the hustlers I watched would use house cues, or cheap brands of cues, to insinuate that they were rookies, that they were raw, unskilled newcomers on the billiards scenes. They would take those cheap cues, and they would make one or two impressive shots, then they would miss all the easy shots.

Their opponents would watch them, and they would focus on the easy shots the hustlers missed, chalk the brilliant shots up to beginner's luck, bet a load of cash, and they would lose.

There were also hustlers who pretended to be drunk or physically impaired. And there were the hustlers who pretended to be crazy and volatile.

Hustling was a form of bullying. And I hate bullying.

I had never hustled anyone before Reilly came calling in 2005. It ran against my moral grain. I knew there was no pleasure in being good, pretending to be bad, and stealing someone's money.

I always played for my winnings legitimately, mostly gambling against men. Every man who walks into a pool hall, after all, thinks he can beat a woman. The only disguise I ever needed was to show up female. I once took $90,000 from a guy too dense to realize that a woman could play pool better than a man.

Two, I was too recognizable. We went to a wig store and a beauty store that sold various things to disguise me. I bought a fake rubber nose, some cheap cat-eye glasses, cheap jewelry, and a matching denim top and pants that were completely different from my style.

Three, How are we going to find a mark, a poor unsuspecting soul, to gamble against the fake me? Although it's hard to feel too bad taking someone's money when you know they were willing to take yours. George said he'd figure that part out. I wondered if this was a good idea. Maybe it would make our sport look bad. Or me. Or maybe our victim wouldn't take being hustled well and we could easily get ourselves in a bind.

But Reilly was a national sports figure and he wanted to write about me. And we were, after all, doing it for journalistic reasons. I knew hustling was a major part of the allure of pool with the American public. That's why *The Hustler* and *The Color of Money* had been so popular at the box office.

I knew those same people would eat this Reilly article up.

> "In her formal marketing plan, I wrote, 'PR til you drop.' Because no matter how big the fish, it doesn't change the size

> of the pond very much. No matter how you cut it, billiards is a niche sport. She couldn't become famous by staying in the niche. We had to get her in the public eye as much as we could."
>
> —Tom George, Lee's longtime manager

I always took advantage of any media opportunities that I got, whether it was with the WPBA, through Octagon, or by networking at every charity or corporate party I attended. I believed the only way I was going to make a good living playing pool was by having sponsors and endorsements. I was only valuable to them if I was influential, and that meant I needed a following. So I did the work. I knew what had to be done and Tom agreed, even when it meant sitting on the phone in the dark, late at night, tired and ready to fall asleep, talking to a sports radio station in Dubuque, Iowa, at 11:00 PM.

There were probably 17 listeners hearing what I had to say about cues, composure, and being an icon of the sport. But I called in to that radio station at 11:00 PM in Iowa, because that's what I believed it took to build my following. I couldn't think about the end result. If I thought about odds, I would've never become No. 1. If I thought about odds, I would've never become known as The Black Widow of Billiards.

Tom would take me to Radio Row at the Super Bowl each year, and I would do 20 to 25 interviews in one afternoon. I was willing to do whatever it took to promote The Black Widow brand.

So, when Reilly came calling, I did what I was supposed to do and, reluctantly, I said yes.

I spent the day of our hustle disguising myself and, when I looked in the mirror, even I was shocked at the transformation I saw. I was no longer The Black Widow. I was a 33-year-old nobody off the streets. I thought, this could be really fun, or it could turn very ugly.

> "The Black Widow is to pool what Ben Franklin is to kites, Wallenda is to heights, and Google is to sites. Her ink-black Rapunzel hair, Asian beauty, and killer stroke make her the most famous player in the world. So, why doesn't anybody in this Indianapolis pool hall recognize her?"
>
> —Rick Reilly,
> in his 2005 *Sports Illustrated* article on Lee,
> "Doing the Hustle."

I was a household name in 2005, recognized just about anywhere I went, and I was regularly making appearances on TV. During the hustle, my slender, 5'9" body was morphed into a voluptuous, curvy figure.

My cohort, Reilly, became a guy named "Billy." He wore a white tanktop, a lot of fake gold, and a Navy-blue derby hat, pretending to be a drunk pimp daddy kind of figure. He was acting a little drunk, playing $100 a rack against George, who also acted a bit drunk. They were tossing hundreds of dollars back and forth, even dropping bills on occasion.

My husband, George, a reformed hustler himself, and one of the best players in the world, helped us with our disguises and plan of attack. He was our hustling guru. He promised us that someone would show up that day.

Sure enough, like clockwork, our prey walked in.

> "He's a local shark, and as soon as he hears [by way of George's anonymous call] that there are a couple of drunks, and a hoochie, betting Benjamins over at Claude & Annie's Poolroom, he double-times it straight into the trap."
>
> —Rick Reilly,
> 2005 *Sports Illustrated* article on hustling with Lee

Our opponent was a local furniture salesman named Jim Calder. He unpacked his cue and asked if we wanted to play for a little money. Of course we did.

It started with a $100, 9-ball bet against George. As they played, I was at the table next to them, and I was banging balls like a novice. I stuck my butt out and struck the balls clumsily; I probably should have won an Oscar for that performance.

My fake nose started peeling off as I played and I had to keep pushing the rubber back into place. The diaper pads stuffed into my pants for my exaggerated butt was slowly sliding down my legs and I had to hoist them up. I put on this amazing act, and Calder fell for it.

"Hell, let's play for some real money," George said to Calder. "How about you play our girl here?"

Calder looked at me and said to George, "No, sorry. I don't play women."

George said, "Okay, well, I guess we're done with you then." He racked the balls and started playing Reilly again, now for $300 a game. Calder didn't want to play me, but he'd lost two games to George in what looked like lucky fashion. He was stuck $200 down and he really wanted to win his money back, but the guys refused to play him again. His greed finally got the best of him.

"Alright, I'll play her," Calder said.

George replied, "Well she's not as good as you, so you're going to need to spot her the 7-ball," meaning, I could win by making the 7-ball or the 9-ball in a legal shot, but Calder could only win by making the 9-ball. Calder quickly agreed. From what he saw, he could spot me much more than that. He was a known, local gambler, a particularly good player. Then George said, "And you gotta give us odds on the money. How much do you have in your pocket?" Calder reluctantly emptied his pockets and counted out $700 and some change. George said, "So this is what we're going to do. We'll bet our $500 against all the money in your pocket for one game of 9-ball.

Calder said, "No way. We've got to play a race to nine. One game could get too lucky."

Rick said, "Hey buddy, we were having ourselves a good time til you came around. We don't need you. Make it a race to three, take it or leave it. We can't be here all day." After a moment, Calder relented. Reilly said, "Hey, baby girl, you gonna make big daddy some money today?"

I rolled my eyes at him with a smile and lit my cigarette. "Don't I always?"

"Sometimes you'd kill for a video camera, the No. 4-ranked women's player in the world itching herself with her cue, primping in the window, and holding the stick like a nail file," Reilly wrote in his article. "She tries to throw the first game, but the mark scratches on the 9-ball."

In the second game, I buried balls like a pro into the pocket, and then I missed on purpose, only to make sure I left Calder blocked. I won.

> "Now the pigeon is frying. He's got $700 riding on the third game, and this hoochie is getting luckier than Paris Hilton's chihuahua. Now she combos the 1 into the 9, sending the 9 off the far cushion and back the entire length of the table into the corner pocket."
>
> —Rick Reilly, in his 2005 *Sports Illustrated* article

"Yo, Billieeeee!" I screeched, still playing my hoochie role. "So, like, I win, right?"

The hustle was over.

As Calder raged, furious he'd lost $700 to some no-name woman off the streets, George turned to him, "Double or nothing?"

I pinched Reilly really hard on his side and whispered to him, "We have to let this guy off the hook now."

Reilly called me a party pooper, but he agreed.

As Calder walked up to pay what he owed us, Reilly put his arm around me and asked him, "Do you know who this is?" Calder did not. "Take a good look at her," Reilly told him. Still nothing.

"Babe, do your thing," Reilly said to me. I opened up my pants, and I started pulling out the pads. I took off my sunglasses, I ripped off my wig, and my long hair fell out.

Calder knew then. He put his head down and said, "You're The Black Widow."

I laughed as Reilly gave him back his $700 and called him a good sport, saying, "A lot of guys would have cracked the bridge over somebody's skull for this."

"Are you kidding?" he said, "I just got hustled by The Black Widow. This is a story that I'll be able to tell my kids and grandkids."

No one got hurt. Calder was happy, Rick was happy, everyone was happy. We walked away triumphant, laughing about the ruse we had just pulled off. We could not have scripted it any better. Everything had gone perfectly.

The Rick Reilly episode gave me national exposure, and it taught Calder something I already knew. Be careful when you are hustling someone, because you might be the one being hustled.

And, in life, you really never know what is going to be thrown your way, or what you might have to overcome.

CHAPTER 24

WHEN THE DEMONS COME FOR YOU, NEVER GIVE UP

THE MOST BEAUTIFUL, inspiring, and emotional words I have ever read in my life were spoken more than a century ago by president Theodore Roosevelt. Those words have become my life's anthem. Those words are *my* quote, the quote that pushed me through as I fought the naysayers and struggled through the darkness.

I have always kept these words in my heart and in my soul. From the days I was working my butt off to become the No. 1 pool player in the world to now, as I fight for my life, I have repeated Roosevelt's words a million times and, yet, I still get emotional every single time.

This quote touches me so very deeply. It has given me so much strength through the years. It is like Roosevelt wrote these words in 1910 just for me.

> "It is not the critic who counts, not the man who points out how the strong man stumbles, or where the doer of deeds could have done better. The credit belongs to the man who is actually in the arena, whose face is marred by dust and sweat and blood, who strives valiantly, who errs and comes up short again and again, because there is no effort without error or shortcoming, but who knows the great enthusiasms, the great devotions, who spends himself in a worthy cause; who, at the best, knows, in the end, the triumph of high achievement, and who, at the worst, if he fails, at least he fails while daring greatly, so that his place shall never be with those cold and timid souls who knew neither victory nor defeat."

Throughout my life, it has taken me so much strength and courage not to quit. There have been so many people out there, on the sidelines, ready to point the finger and criticize. The local women players, billiard room owners, the gamblers, the media, billiards industry leaders, the veteran women of the WPBA, and fans of the game; this quote reminded me that it really doesn't really matter what they think. I was the one who was daring to compete. I was the one that was putting myself out there.

For so many years, I felt like I was so unlucky. Everything I wanted was not meant to be. But I was so addicted to pool, I just couldn't quit. I knew the odds were against me ever achieving my dreams but it just didn't matter. I could only focus on today. What I could do today to be the change I want to see in the world. I was always trying to persist and I was always trying to give my very best effort, despite the obstacles trying to stop me every step of the way. Some of those obstacles were, admittedly, self-created, and some were out of my control.

Even after becoming the No. 1 women's pool player in the world, I fought demons, I fought insecurities, I fought pain, and I fought haters.

Throughout my career, I had plenty of failures, and many really dismal, dark days as I tried to forge ahead. But I also had plenty of victories and successes, which always kept me going, kept my spirit alive, and made me realize I could persevere even when the most dire odds were against me.

As I rose above the ashes, time and time again, I always felt a sense of sweet revenge. Not revenge against anyone in particular, just revenge against what sometimes could be a cruel world.

But none of those moments of perseverance, of turning hopeless failure into glorious success, could ever hold a candle to one of the proudest moments of my career, when I overcame the insurmountable and rose to the top in glorious victory.

It was 1999 and I was in my late twenties, competing in the WPBA Gentleman Jack Dallas Shootout in Texas. It was the last day of the tournament, and I had made it to the quarterfinals. I was standing at the tournament desk, looking over the schedule, surrounded by other players and the tournament director.

It was almost time for my match to be called and I was more than ready. I was pumped up. I was going to win this whole damn thing. I'd been practicing a lot with my coach, Bob, doing drills, refining my stroke and my preshot routine, as well as doing strength training to support my back. We'd worked it out that I would play for an hour, then rest and lay back for 20 minutes.

But my evil back had other ideas. It decided to fail on me right then and there. Out of nowhere, I got a horrible, deep stab of pain through my spine and I fell to the ground.

As I laid on the hard floor, I looked up at all those people hovering over me and I screamed out, "Oh no! No! No! My back!" I was truly freaking out. I started crying and trembling; I was in excruciating pain.

Unless you have experienced severe scoliosis, there's no way to really grasp or explain the pain and helplessness that comes with the disease. When my back would go into spasms or lock up or exude relentless pain, it was never just my back that was the problem. It was almost like I lost all strength and control of my limbs, too. Scoliosis was often a cruel invasion of my entire body. A lot of times, when I get severe back spasms, my legs get so weak that I can't really walk.

Lying on the floor, set to play in the quarterfinals at the Dallas Shootout, I cursed myself. *Why didn't you just have the surgery? Why did you have to be so stubborn?*

Despite the intense, uncontrollable pain I had endured as an elite billiards player, I had always fought the doctors tooth and nail to never have surgery again. I'd had plenty of opportunities and had been told plenty of times that the surgeons could help me.

But I had been through that horrifying back surgery when I was 13 years old, when I was initially diagnosed with scoliosis, and I couldn't imagine going through the suffering and the misery I felt in 1984. There was no chance I would do that again. I always said to anyone who would listen, "Another surgery? Kill me first."

Now here I was, fifteen years past my only surgery. At the time, I was trying to survive on a transcutaneous electrical nerve stimulation (TENS) unit, a battery-operated device that delivered small electrical impulses through electrodes to invade my nervous system, reducing its ability to transmit pain signals to the spinal cord and brain.

I was also eating Advil like there was no tomorrow. And I was on Vioxx, a prescription medicine used for arthritis and acute pain in adults. I was using heating pads and massage belts. I was trying anything, other than surgery, to ward off the pain.

But none of that was working in 1999. I was on the ground and I was too weak to walk. My coach, Bob Carman, was there, along with a few friends. I remember them bending down slowly to carefully pick me up. Bob and I had not been working together for that long and he was really unsure if he should listen to me and bring me to the lounge or send me to the hospital. As he lifted me, I started crying out, "Ow, ow, ow! You're hurting me." He put me down and apologized, but now didn't know what to do.

"I'm so sorry," he said. "Did I hurt your back?"

"No, Bob. You're stepping on my hair!"

Thankfully, he worked it out and I was carried down the hall to the ladies' lounge. Thank God, it was a posh lounge with soft carpet, cushy loveseats, and a coffee table.

Still, I was lying on a carpeted floor where people walked with their dirty shoes, and I had my legs up in the air, trying to soothe the pain. It was embarrassing. I asked for someone to bring me a chair, not a soft loveseat, but a harder chair to try to take the pressure off my lower back.

I remember the chair being delivered, I remember Bob handing me a pill for the pain, and I remember asking for a phone. I was in a panic. I knew my match would be announced any minute, with a 15-minute grace period to get to the match before it would be called as a forfeit. George and I had been married three years at the point, and I still thought of him as my hero. This was the first time in my life where my back was against the wall and I called for help. He picked up the phone, and said, "Hey babe. What's up?"

I almost broke into tears just hearing his voice. I told George that it was the final day of the tournament and I wasn't even able to stand. My spine was pulsing. I was on the floor of the bathroom. I didn't know what to do. My legs had a tendency to get really weak when my back went out. I wasn't sure if I'd even be able to walk.

I didn't know what advice George would give, but I definitely didn't expect him to say what he did.

"I'm proud of you. I'm sure you tried your best, but why don't you just go ahead and come on home," he said on our phone call. "Just take the forfeit, go upstairs, rest, catch a flight tomorrow, then you'll recover, and you'll do better next time."

George told me playing the rest of this tournament wasn't worth the permanent risk to my back. It wasn't worth the pain and it wasn't worth the pressure.

I couldn't believe what I was hearing. I was really pissed. What was the point of marrying a fellow pro pool player if not to have his understanding of what it was like to want to rule the green felt table?

Quit? I wasn't going to quit.

"What?! Are you kidding? Are you serious?" I said to George. "There's no way in hell I'm just giving up in a forfeit. They're going to have to grab that trophy and curl it out of my bloody, dead hands. They're going to have to beat me, and they're going to have to lift me off the felt."

George knew me so well that he was expecting that response from me, and he had his own retort.

"Okay, Jeanette. If you're going to stay and play and risk damage to your body and put yourself through more pain, when you could be resting in your hotel room, then you better hella win," George said. "If you can bend down to miss that ball, then you can be damn sure you can bend down to *make* that ball."

Yes. Yes. Yes. That's exactly what I wanted to hear from George. I picked myself up off the floor and, with help from other players, I hobbled to the tournament room.

> "The 1999 WPBA Gentleman Jack Dallas Shootout was neither the most prestigious nor lucrative title Jeanette Lee ever won. But it is definitely one of the most memorable for The Black Widow. On the final day of the tournament, Lee won

> four matches while struggling with paralyzing back spasms that almost forced her to forfeit."
>
> —*Billiards Digest*,
> "The Agony of Victory: Lee Strains to Top Corr,"
> February 1999

During each match, every time I bent down for a shot, I would focus completely on that shot. I had to take this one shot at a time. My arms were shaking, and the teardrops were falling on the table.

Some of the people there thought I was crying because I felt sorry for myself. I was crying because of the pain. The pain was so loud. Still, nearly 25 years later, I don't know how to explain it. I know pain is not a sound, but my back was screaming. The pain permeated my entire body, making me so very weak.

Between shots, I used my cue stick as a cane, and I used the rail for balance as I walked around the table. Somehow, I managed to beat Line Kjørsvik, Gerda Hofstätter, and Allison Fisher to make it to the finals. I told myself to keep hanging on, to keep fighting.

In the final match, I faced Karen Corr, a WPBA newcomer. She came on strong, taking the first four racks in the race-to-11 set. But then I took seven straight games, at times having to walk away from the table because of the intense pain.

At one point, I had to sit down. A fan poured me a glass of water and helped me get settled into a chair. I sat there as the pain begged me to forfeit. It was telling me to forfeit. I willed myself not to give up, and I didn't.

As the match resumed, Corr fought back to a 7–7 tie, but then I pulled ahead 10–8.

> "With ball-in-hand, after Corr scratched on the break, Lee gently worked her way to a 4–9 combination. 'Please let me

> make this ball,' she said as she lined up the title clincher. She dropped the 9, then buried her face in her hands and cried."
>
> —*Billiards Digest*, February 1999

I vividly remember making that last ball fall into the pocket at the Dallas Shootout. I had my back to the crowd and, after I made the winning shot, I turned around to face them. And that crowd went ballistic. Those people went crazy.

Throughout the day of the finals, the fans in Dallas had been rooting for me, rooting for this underdog who shouldn't have been the underdog. They were rooting for a woman who, by no fault of her own, was struggling in pain. Whenever I needed a boost of energy throughout that tournament, the fans came through.

Now they were rejoicing in my unlikely victory.

As I turned around toward the crowd and smiled, I couldn't keep that smile on my face for long. I tried so hard to be positive, but I couldn't believe I had won this Dallas Shootout, that I had overcome the pain no one in that room could ever understand.

I started bawling like a baby. It was the first and the last time I ever cried after a match. There was so much adrenaline pumping through my body, and so much relief. These were tears, not from pain, but from victory—and relief that it was over.

But as that glorious moment faded, the pain quickly worsened. I laid in my hotel room in agony. And more pain followed, year after year, as I endured countless surgeries, even as I continued to be a billiards superstar.

Then 20 years after the Dallas Shootout, I felt a kind of pain I had never faced. It was the worst pain I had ever felt in my life, the kind of pain that tortures not just your body, but your mind.

It was the pain of Stage 4 ovarian cancer.

It is not the critic who counts, not the man who points out how the strong man stumbles, or where the doer of deeds could have done better. The credit belongs to the man who is actually in the arena, whose face is marred by dust and sweat and blood, who strives valiantly...

Those words, spoken by Roosevelt more than 110 years ago, resonated with me again as I fought terminal cancer, as I once again tried to rise above the ashes, as I tried to conquer the demons, and as I relied on family and friends more than ever.

I also turned to the one constant that has been with me all my life, the one relationship that never bailed on me. My faith in God.

CHAPTER 25

FINALLY GRASPING WHAT IT MEANS TO BE A CHRISTIAN

I OWE SO MUCH IN MY LIFE TO GOD and my Christianity. My faith has carried me through some incredibly tough times. No matter what stage I was at in my life, from being a lost rebellious teenager to becoming a pool sensation, I never lost my faith.

I may have turned away from it a time or two, or tried to put blinders on, so I didn't have to think about God watching what I was doing. But I always believed in God.

At the toughest times in my life, I would yell out to God, furious, screaming, and shaking my fists. My mom would say, "Jeanette, why don't you believe in God and his plan?"

I did believe in God. Of course, I did. If I didn't, why would I even be talking to him? No one yells at a person they don't believe is real.

I not only believed God was real but, through the years, God has been the one true constant in my life, the one person I could turn to, who was never too busy or working too hard or too jealous of me or too good for me. I often felt Him listening when I prayed to Him for answers, and when I didn't, I could flip the Bible open to any page and miraculously, there in front of me was my answer. I learned this trick when I was quite young. The Bible is always a source of strength when things get too overwhelming for me to handle. I'm such a control freak that I would always try to handle things on my own and mainly just praised God, thanked God, and asked him to bless my family and friends. I asked Him to help me stay true to Him, be a good example to others, and strengthen my faith. But when there was a job to be done, I would handle it by myself. Until I couldn't. Then I would get on my hands and knees and cry. I'd always wonder why it was so hard for me to lean into God when my life got shaky.

But I have to be honest, our relationship has ebbed and flowed. And there have been times when I have been really down on Christianity.

I have been to many churches in my life and, at those churches, I have met some really great people. But I also have met some really fake people, some hypocritical people, and some judgmental people. I would look at those people being gossipy or selfish or rude and think to myself, "Really? What hypocrites! I can't believe they have the nerve to judge me and then call themselves Christians?"

I absolutely hated the hypocrisy. How can you call yourself a Christian when you spend so much time gossiping and hurting others? I carried resentment toward them for years. I find it strange—though perhaps more common than you'd think—that even though I was hurt by both Christians and non-Christians, I found myself judging the Christians more harshly. Why? I think it's because I had a preconceived expectation that by calling themselves Christians, they had a responsibility to act more like Jesus Christ and not act like blatant gossipy sinners. They shouldn't continuously, knowingly, say and do things that work against what scriptures tell us to do. Leviticus 19:18

says, "Do not seek revenge or bear a grudge against a fellow Israelite, but love your neighbor as yourself. I am the Lord."

The Lord God is holy, and because we're made in the image of God, those who are called to emulate God's holiness are to do so by acting with mercy and love toward their fellow human beings. Where was their love? What made them think they were better than me? At least I'm not going around judging and gossiping about others.

So here I was, thinking that, as Christians, they shouldn't be judging me. Even if I'm not behaving in a way they approve of, they should be loving me, helping me, teaching and guiding me the right way, not ostracizing me. And yet I later realized, as I was judging those other Christians, I was being a hypocrite myself. On the tour, as the women treated me terribly, I should have been praying for them. Instead, I judged them, and I felt anger and resentment toward them.

Among those women were Loree Jon Jones and Robin Dodson, who were known as very public Christians. Loree Jon had a beautiful voice, and she could bring people to tears as she sang "Amazing Grace." At the morning Bible studies at Billiard Congress of America's open tournaments, Robin and Loree Jon were the first ones there.

I remember thinking what hypocrites they were, how awful they were to me, yet they called themselves Christians. I mumbled underneath my breath, "I don't even know how you can pray at night. How can you even stand yourself."

Here I was, in my mind, the only one of the three of us acting like a true Christian. A few years later, I realized I hadn't been acting Christian at all.

It was at one of those tournaments, around 1:00 or 2:00 AM in the morning, when I heard a knock on my hotel door. I wasn't expecting anyone, so I stayed in bed, figuring the person would go away. But the knocker was persistent and, when I went to open the door, there stood Loree Jon.

She was sobbing.

Through her tears, Loree Jon told me that she had been praying before bed and, while she prayed, I kept coming into her head. She told me she felt convicted in her heart for the way she had treated me, how she had allowed herself to go along with the way the other women on the tour ostracized me.

"Jeanette, I'm just human," Loree Jon said to me. "I've always struggled with getting caught up in gossip. It's not right. I don't want to do it. Sometimes, I catch myself. Sometimes I don't, but I'm sorry. I'm really sorry."

I forgave Loree Jon right there at my hotel room door, and we have been good ever since. A few years later, Robin apologized to me as well. From then on, our relationship developed into true friendship. I have great respect and admiration for both of them. And if I were to catch them gossiping again (which I haven't), I knew to love them, pray for them, and talk to them in a non-judgmental, loving way. They're incredibly good people and they have given me so much strength and encouragement. I value our relationship. What those two women did for me changed my way of thinking about my Christianity forever. Yes, we should hold ourselves to a higher standard as Christians, but that's precisely my point. *We* should hold *ourselves*, and not others, to a higher standard. We should love ourselves as God loves us, and we should love our neighbors as we love ourselves.

Christians are just normal human beings, with difficult flaws and bad habits, who chose to have faith that there is a living God, that Jesus died on the cross to forgive our sins and pay our debts so we could be forgiven and enter the kingdom of Heaven, and that the Holy Spirit lives inside us, guiding us. So some of us choose to believe in Him and we're not afraid to share that with others because our great country allows us to. We're also taught to share fellowship with others Christians and to share the Gospel with nonbelievers so they could be saved also. We are imperfect and we will always be imperfect.

It's easy to get wrapped up in finding imperfections in others when you're hurting, but we're really hurting ourselves more than we're hurting them.

That's not what Christianity is about. It is not about perfection. And, if there are hypocrites in the world, it's not because they're Christians. It's because they're human. That's why we should be keeping our eye on Him and in the Bible and in church and loving unconditionally, and *not* on other people who are also just trying to live their lives well on Earth until we can be with Him again in Heaven, or until they meet their death and wherever their beliefs take them.

Loree Jon and Robin taught me a big life lesson—how important it is not to judge other people, not just for their sake, but for my sake. When you judge people, you put blinders on. You can't see beyond your own disgust. You can't see that maybe that person is struggling, too.

I realized I had no right to judge whether a Christian was being a Christian. We are all human. We are all going to fail. We are going to embarrass ourselves and let other people down. And we are going to, hopefully, realize our mistakes and ask for forgiveness.

To this day, I am so thankful that Loree Jon had the courage to come to my hotel room in the wee hours of the morning all those years ago. It could not have been easy for her to knock on my door and admit she had made a mistake in the way she treated me.

It wasn't easy for me, either, to realize I had made my own mistakes, judging her.

That encounter showed me the goodness of Christianity, the goodness of God, and the importance of keeping my eyes on the Lord and not on judging others. It strengthened my faith and reminded me why my faith mattered more than ever. And all of that has stuck with me in my darkest hours.

CHAPTER 26

LIVING MOMENT BY SWEET MOMENT, ONE DAY AT A TIME

I SHOULDN'T BE SITTING here inside my Tampa home writing this book with the windows open, as the sun streams in and as a warm breeze caresses my face. My daughter Cheyenne shouldn't be lying on the bed next to me, snuggled up to our sweet, tiny, fawn-colored emotional support chihuahua, Thor.

My two younger daughters, Chloe and Savannah, shouldn't be in the other room deciding what to pack for our upcoming trip to Orlando, where we will make amazing, incredible memories, visiting four parks in one week—Universal Studios, Islands of Adventure, Discovery Cove, and Aquatica.

None of these wonderful things should be happening. This book probably should have never been written.

I should not be here. I should be dead.

It's been more than three years since my cancer diagnosis, which doctors told me was incurable and will never be in remission. I've gotten over that dismal reality as best I can. I no longer feel like I'm standing on the edge of a cliff, just waiting for the final nudge that will push me off into eternal darkness.

I've accepted what might be my harsh and sad truth—that my life most likely will be measured in months, and maybe years, rather than decades.

I do not know how much time I have left on this Earth. None of us do, really. But I know my years are probably shorter than most. At least that's what the odds say.

My type of cancer, Stage 4 ovarian cancer, which had already spread throughout my body when it was discovered in January 2021, is pretty much the worst kind of cancer diagnosis a person can get.

Initially, doctors told me I might have just six months to live. In a best-case scenario, I might have a few years. Instead of focusing on any of that, I decided to live moment by sweet moment, one day at a time.

And, miraculously, I kept getting another day, and another day. And then another month, and another month. And I hope another year, and another year, and many more years to come.

I am cautiously optimistic that could happen. And while I don't want this to sound like a pharmaceutical advertisement, or maybe I do, I truly believe there is one drug to thank for keeping me alive. A drug that I believe saved my life.

My bonus time on this Earth—the time cancer patients live past their original prognosis—has a lot to do with Olaparib. Sold under the brand name Lynparza, it is a medication for the maintenance treatment of BRCA-mutated advanced ovarian cancer.

My cancer was so advanced when it was discovered that it was too late for radiation. Lynparza was part of my original cocktail of chemotherapy treatments, which were a brutal and unbearable regimen. I slept a lot. I slept most of my life away during those summer months of 2021 as I went through the chemo.

> "Most of the people who take the regimen Jeanette took can't complete it. They physically can't abide by it. But it was the only real chance she had. And she did it."
>
> —Don Wardell,
> Lee's longtime physician and friend

For people who finish the type of chemo I went through, the average life expectancy is two years. I'm nearing what doctors call a "remarkable three years." I still take Lynparza daily, now for maintenance, and I give that drug full credit for saving my life, at least in the short term.

My scans have been cancer free for the past two years, but that doesn't mean I'm in remission. My cancer is the kind that likes to return. I know it's lurking somewhere inside of my body, ready to attack whenever it decides it wants to strike again. This disease is insidious but, for now, doctors can't measure it.

And that means I am beating the odds once again. But beating the odds, I know very well, has never been easy.

I am much weaker and much more fatigued than I have ever been in my life, and my doctors are pleading with me to gain weight.

During the chemo treatments, I reached my highest weight, 152 pounds. But for the past two years, my body has dwindled, at some points, to scary lows. I've been fighting to keep my weight up, eating whatever sounds good to me and whatever I can force myself to swallow.

Some days it's chicken and rice, or salmon and broccoli, or a BLT sandwich, or a couple of take-out sushi rolls. Sometimes it's a healthy salad, but some days all I can get down are the protein shakes. I'm supposed to be drinking at least two of those a day, in addition to my meals.

Last year, at a doctor's appointment, I stepped on the scale, and I weighed in at 113 pounds. On my 5-foot-9-inch frame, that is on the level of a near skeleton. When I saw that number flashing, it really shook me. I thought I had been eating enough. I thought I was doing what I was supposed to be doing.

Doctors tell me it's dangerous to be that skinny. Stage 4 cancer is a wicked opponent. If I don't gain weight, my doctors tell me, I won't be able to fight off the cancer if it returns. And I will die.

My doctors are always telling me, "You must eat at least three meals a day, Jeanette." But sometimes my body aches so badly that all I want to do is go to bed. Some evenings, by 6:00 PM, I have taken all my night medicines and crawled into bed, skipping dinner. And then, there are the mornings when I wake up and I feel like I can't face the day.

I open my eyes and I think about what's in front of me, the pain and the sadness, and sometimes the depression. I close my eyes, go back to sleep, and I don't wake up until 11:00 AM, missing breakfast. Some days, the only meal I eat is lunch.

Before the cancer, I used to cook all the time, making delicious, spicy, Korean cuisine and Italian food. Now, all I do is warm up food that is already cooked, or I pull something out of the freezer and pop it into the microwave. My family and friends are always trying to help me out, bringing over homemade sweets and baked casseroles. One of my daughter's teachers, a trained chef, brought over a giant tub of chicken fettuccine alfredo, shrimp scampi, basil pesto pasta, and a beautiful Caesar salad after a surgery. It was incredibly thoughtful.

I try to eat, and I try my absolute hardest to stay positive. I have to be positive for my daughters. But it is not easy. Sometimes, I feel very alone.

I never really talked to anyone about my cancer on a deep level. Due to COVID-19, I never went to a psychologist or a therapist to work through my diagnosis. I never joined a cancer support group (though I have now). A lot of the time, I am inside my own head, which means sometimes I feel like I'm on an emotional downward spiral.

My memory and comprehension have taken a hit, which is really frustrating to me, and that has slowly cut away at my self-esteem. It's discouraging, because I have so many things I still want to do in life.

These last few years have been very hard on my family, too. I have gone through a roller coaster of mood swings, and I have not been able to be fully present much of the time. I couldn't be there for my daughters the way I wanted to be there for them—helping them with homework, going to the mall to shop, getting our nails done, or just sitting around and talking about life.

Even now, as I try to move on, there are still times I find myself shutting down. I desperately want to be that strong, positive force I used to be. I want to be The Black Widow again. But sometimes that is very hard, when all I want to do is lie in bed with the lights turned off.

I am proud of myself that, despite the health battles I face, I have forced myself to get out and live life. Just months after finishing my chemo treatments, my friends Jeannie Seaver and Sonya Chbeeb invited me to an open tournament.

I returned to professional pool action, competing in the Diamond Open in Aiken, South Carolina, where fellow players literally broke down in tears at the mere sight of me.

One of those players was Allison Fisher who, through the years, had been my biggest nemesis. She talked about how grateful she was to see me back at the table. I met Allison in the quarterfinals of the tournament.

> "Aside from a frailty of movement, an indication of some struggles with pain, Lee competed with all the verve and skills that have been a part of her game for as long as she's been carrying the moniker of the deadly Black Widow."
>
> —*AZBilliards.com*,
> "Fisher Downs The Black Widow in Winners' Side Quarterfinal," October 2021

During the match, I had virtually no unforced errors and, though I didn't win, I finished in the money. It was an unexplainable, sweet victory for me. My hair was gone, my body was weak, but I had proven I could still compete with one of the top women in the world.

Since that tournament, I have made other appearances. I have traveled for the American Poolplayers Association and, in December 2022, my ESPN documentary *Jeanette Lee Vs.* debuted. That was an emotional, full-circle moment for my career. ESPN, after all, is the network that launched me into billiards stardom.

People often ask me why I feel the need to go out and compete, when my body is fighting a ruthless disease. They insinuate that maybe I should hang up my cue and leave the sport of pool behind.

Why am I playing again? That answer is very easy for me. I still play because I love the game. I'm never going to stop loving the game. I know I can get better than I am. I just need to make the time to muster up the strength to practice. I need to be more disciplined.

Sometimes, I dream of going back on the tour. I want to go back on the tour, but my manager, Tom George, has helped to keep me grounded.

When I was diagnosed with cancer, Tom and I sat down and we made a list of my priorities. Priority No. 1 was to focus on my health and well-being, doing everything I could to stay alive. Priority No. 2 was to focus on spending time with my daughters, making precious memories they could hold on to forever.

My commercial appearances and outings, which help me earn money for my family, came next. Going back on the tour quickly fell to the bottom of the list.

Tom tells me I have done everything I need to do in this sport, that I don't have anything to prove anymore. To be honest, I'm not trying to prove anything. I never played pool for fame. I didn't do it for the money. It wasn't about any of that. I just wanted to improve my game and compete, compete, *compete*. It was always about the love of the game.

But deep down in my soul, I know Tom is right. I know the priorities he helped me set as I battle terminal cancer are the right priorities. I've watched the top women today and, compared to five years ago or 10 years ago, they are better, and they are stronger. It would take a lot of practicing and a lot of hard work for me to get up to their level.

And the amount of time it would take me to get to that level would be a full-time job, at least 50 or 60 hours a week. I'm not willing to give that up, that time I could be spending with my daughters.

In a way, that makes me very sad, the thought of never being on the pro women's circuit again. I often find myself in and out of depression, but there is also a side of me that fights to keep going. I plan to live a long time. I can't let the setbacks in my life defeat me. I have to stay positive.

In 2023, I was presented with the APA's Achievement Through Adversity Award at the league's operator convention. The award, which honors billiards personalities who have overcome significant adversity to achieve success, meant so much to me.

> "Today, we are honored to have with us a woman who has exemplified this quality her entire life, whether battling her own body, her surroundings, or an opponent on the pool table. Jeanette Lee has time and time again found a way to overcome tremendous odds, while building her own global brand. We are honored to have her with us today, and blessed to be able to call her one of our own."
>
> —Jason Bowman,
> introducing Lee for her 2023 APA award

I went to the podium and I told my story, how God had grounded me two years before with a terminal cancer diagnosis. That diagnosis made me stop and take a look at my life. And everywhere I turned, all around me, were blessings.

"All of you guys, I just love you. That's it. I'm very thankful, and if you guys are ever going through anything, I can say, from my own perspective, know you are not alone," I told the crowd. "It's the ones that have gone through things and made it to the other side. They are the ones with the voice to make a change, to be the change you want to see in the world."

I had learned early on from my mother and my experience of later becoming the national spokesperson for the Scoliosis Association, Inc., that everything I went through in my life meant something, that the struggles I faced had a greater purpose. And I always wanted to do something good with that.

I have a plaque hanging on the wall next to the door that leads out of my house. On that plaque are three simple words: *No Matter What.*

No matter what happens, I must always forge ahead. No matter what comes my way, I must persevere. I tell my girls that. I will always love my girls unconditionally, *no matter what!* No matter what happens, we must always forge ahead. I tell my girls that no matter what comes our way, we must persevere, and never give up on ourselves and our dreams, because that is the only way we will ever learn the great plans God has for us. That is the only way we can ever realize our potential and how capable we truly are. But above all, it means that I will always love my girls unconditionally.

Having faith is so important. To know that despite our fears and anxieties, we can overcome more than we ever imagined. We should never live our lives or make decisions based on how we feel. Feelings can deceive us. We can feel like we're drowning or too weak, but the truth of the matter is that strength and courage is not in the absence of fear, but in the face of it. When everything is tearing you down and you feel like you can't get up, you can't take another *anything*, and yet you still manage to get out of bed. Put one foot down after another. Wash your face, even though you don't even want to look at yourself in the mirror. Courage isn't waking up and having no doubts, it's getting up when you're positive that you can't. *That* is true courage. And if you do, promise me something. Promise me that you'll take the time to be proud of yourself.

You are stronger than you believe. Always remember, you don't have to feel strong to be strong. You just have to keep going. And you can do it. I believe in you. You are stronger than you believe.

Trust me.

CHAPTER 27

WRITING YOUR OWN STORY IS THE HARDEST THING TO DO

WHEN I VISIT MY PARENTS IN NEW YORK CITY, we sometimes sit on the couch together and we flip through the worn, plastic-covered pages of our old family photo albums. Sometimes, I break down in tears, looking at that young, skinny, Korean girl who was always insecure, always scared, and always intimidated.

I see the smile on her face in all the photos. But I know that, sometimes, that smile was a façade. I see a girl who is trying to be brave and strong, but I know, most of the time, she was faking her way through all of that.

I look at the photo of me at five years old in a dark blue swimsuit with my hands on my hips, looking fierce. I look at the photo of me and my sister, Doris, twirling Hula-Hoops, and I can see, even in that still shot, the look of admiration I have on my face for Doris. The look of wanting to be able to spin that hoop as magically as she could spin the hoop, and of always wanting to be more like my older sister.

There are photos of me at nine, 10, and 11 years old on the playground, and in sports, trying to destroy the boys. There is a photo of me lying in a hospital bed at 13, after my scoliosis surgery. I was screaming in pain on the inside, but I was so drugged up, I couldn't get the screams out. I can see the look of fear on my face.

There is a photo of me stuffed into a big, clunky brace, the contraption I had to wear in middle school to make sure my spine stayed in place after the surgery. I look into my eyes in that picture and I see the horror I felt wearing that brace, how it made me feel like a monster.

There are photos of me with piercings, wearing cut-up, fringed, camo vests during my rebellious teenage years. I look like a badass in the photos, but I know that underneath I was nothing more than a lonely young woman who wanted to fit in, and who was desperate to find acceptance.

Scattered all throughout the album are photos of me with my mom and my dad. But none of those photos show any type of really joyous, loving, close relationship. We almost look like robots in the pictures. I don't remember spending much time with my parents growing up. They were always working.

I know they loved me. I know they always only wanted the best for me. I know I made my mother suffer as I took a road she hadn't planned for me. I know I hurt her deeply when I ran away, and yelled awful, piercing, stinging words at her.

To this day, in my early fifties, I still feel like a little girl sometimes. And it still breaks my heart what I put my parents through. I love my mom and dad dearly, and I am so grateful and blessed that we have been able to heal old wounds and become close.

When I was diagnosed with cancer, I watched my mother start to cry. It was a quiet, gentle sobbing, a cry of helplessness.

> "It's been my honor to be her mother. I am so proud of her, and I love her. I hope we will be together in Heaven someday, and be at peace. I love you."
>
> —Sonja Lee, Jeanette's mother, after her daughter's cancer diagnosis

All I ever wanted to be in this life was a good person. Yes, I wanted to annihilate people at the pool table, but I also wanted to empower other women, be an inspiration to people all over the world, and prove that no matter how far you fall to rock bottom, there is a way to climb back up to the top.

What matters most to me in life has never changed. What matters most to me is family. My parents, my sisters, my extended family, and my children. They will forever be the most precious gifts I have.

When it came time to write my memoir, as terminal cancer put a deadline on my life, I was terrified.

How do you sum up your entire life in one book? How do you make it mean something? How do you make sure you remember all the people who were there for you, all the amazing moments that changed you, all the terrible moments that shaped you, and all the incredible moments you wouldn't trade, even if it meant more time on this Earth?

All I wanted was for this memoir to be inspiring to you, to my fans. And to people who weren't my fans, but who picked up my book not knowing they even wanted to read it, I hope you became captivated, energized, and galvanized to forge ahead in what we all know is never an easy life, but one that is most definitely worth living.

Writing a memoir is like giving a hall of fame speech on steroids. It also sometimes feels like writing your own obituary.

That obituary, my obituary, would read that, aside from my faith, my family, and my friends, the most important thing to me has always been the sport of billiards. It was what took me from a broken human being to a person who felt like she could be good at something, like she could be a hero, like she could be loved.

I found a second family in those pool halls where I played every night, and I found acceptance in the billiards community. And, because of that, I always wanted to be the biggest advocate for my beloved sport.

Throughout my career, people always talked about how I transcended billiards into mainstream media, and how I secured lucrative deals outside of pool. But less talked about was how deeply devoted I was inside the pool industry, how I was one of its biggest allies.

I have been with several of the major billiards equipment manufacturer, including Imperial Billiards, Predator, McDermott, and Escalade Sports. I did countless infomercials for those brands. I also had a long-term column called "Dear Jeanette" which was published in *Billiards Digest.* I showed up for any billiards appearance I could physically be at.

I always wanted desperately to raise billiards from a niche sport to a game as popular as basketball, football, or baseball. Of course, that didn't happen, but I always hoped my time in the sport would shine a light that elevated the game to something people took notice of.

> "Who is the biggest star of the group? It's still Jeanette. Thirty-five years after she first picked up a cue stick, and 15 years after she was done playing competitively, it's still her. And that is winning."
>
> —Tom George, Lee's longtime manager

The shining star inside the billiards industry has been my relationship with the American Poolplayers Association, who promoted me like I was the Taylor Swift of the sport. They not only helped me during the wonderful times of my career, but they helped me during the really dark times.

The APA has been my biggest ally throughout my cancer fight, paying me a salary, even when they didn't have to, when I wasn't doing anything to make money for them. They also helped boost my GoFundMe campaign, which raised hundreds of thousands of dollars for my daughters.

The APA didn't have to do any of that. They did it because they cared about me. Jason Bowman and Greg Fletcher will always be my own personal saviors. After my ESPN documentary *Jeanette Lee Vs.* debuted, the APA immediately aired a podcast, trying to stoke interest in my documentary among the billiards-loving community.

In turn, I am still trying to do all I can for the game, and for the APA, even though I am sometimes so tired, and sometimes in so much pain.

> "Even a couple months ago, she was talking about a fund-raiser and talking about, even if she's not earning money, how she still loves the game, because the game is beautiful, and she still wants to promote the game."
>
> —Doris Lee, Jeanette's sister

Looking back over my life and career, I often wonder, did I do enough? Did I do enough to help people inside and outside of the billiards community? Will people remember me as a kind soul who wasn't putting on an act, who really wanted to make a difference in people's lives?

When I would stay late to sign autographs for fans after playing a grueling match, and as I took young players under my wings, I always wanted them to know that I truly cared about each and every one of them. They weren't just random fans I had met. They were people to me.

I would often go out of my way to make an impact. I always wanted to touch people, especially people who battled scoliosis. I knew the agony of fighting that disease.

One year when my friend and fellow pool player, Stu Mattana, visited me in Indiana, I picked him up at the airport to head back to my house to drop off his things before we went to play pool. Stu and I loved to play straight pool. Those games are usually a race to 100, but we would play races to 500 and 1,000. We were fanatics.

On the way home from the airport, I asked Stu if we could make a quick stop at the hospital. I wanted to visit a young girl who had scoliosis, and her parents, to give them support and encouragement for the surgery she was about to have.

Stu, of course, said yes. He asked me how I knew that family. I told him I didn't know them at all. I had just heard about this girl, and I wanted to bring her family comfort.

> "It was really special to see Jeanette go out of her way to help a family she didn't know, for no real reason, other than to do good. There are a lot of nice pros, but not a lot who would do that."
>
> —Stu Mattana, Lee's longtime friend

I always tried to support every single scoliosis patient and family I was ever made aware of, to be there for them. I remembered, after all, when I was diagnosed with scoliosis and could not see through the darkness to any light.

I remembered lying in my bed after surgery in agony, after doctors had literally broken my spine into pieces.

My mom would put her hands on me and pray. She would say, "Jeanette, God has such a great plan for you. Just trust in him. Lean on God." That made me furious. I would tell my mom to shut up. There was no way she could understand what this felt like.

But then years later, I realized my mom was right all along. My scoliosis happened for a reason. God did have a greater plan for me. I could not have imagined at 13 years old when I was going through all that hell that something good could come from it. But something amazing came from it.

I got to touch thousands of people dealing with scoliosis.

When I first started making a name for myself in pool, my then-manager Sheri asked me to pick a cause, a charity, or some nonprofit agency to support. I knew immediately that I wanted to find a way to support people battling scoliosis.

I found a fairly small organization called The Scoliosis Association, Inc., whose focus was to support the patients and their families, to be there for them, inform them, to find them local support groups, to prepare them for scoliosis, and life after scoliosis.

That was something I never had as I battled the disease. In the early 1980s, I would've never dreamt of something like that. A resource like that just wasn't available. I knew as soon as I talked to the people at The Scoliosis Association, Inc., that this was my calling. This was the one. I loved everything about their mission. I didn't care that they were small.

I took a seat on their board and also became their national spokesperson, which entailed traveling to medical conferences to speak publicly to hundreds of kids about my journey and how I overcame this debilitating disease to pursue my dreams. It was so gratifying to experience the goodness that came from my horrifying experience with scoliosis. Had I stayed a victim by feeling sorry for myself and quitting, I would've never realized the opportunity that I had to inspire others and keep them from suffering alone like I did.

I had no prior experience planning a major fundraiser, but that's what I did. I researched online and studied how to plan fundraisers and I contacted an event planner for a local charity in Indianapolis called Mickey's Camp and asked her tons of questions to get her advice and insight, along with giving me access to the sponsors she had acquired for her camp. I also reached out to billiard companies as well as local restaurants and stores. I put together my first press release copying from ones I obtained online. My first scoliosis event was wildly successful. It was held at Chalkies Billiards in Indianapolis, and we got big-name athletes like Indiana Pacers star Reggie Miller and Indianapolis Colts players Edgerrin James and Marvin Harrison to stop by.

Local radio personalities Bob Kevoian and Tom Griswold, of the nationally syndicated *The Bob & Tom Show*, were there. After that charity, I continued to be a fierce advocate for the small nonprofit.

That is one of my proudest achievements in my life, and there have been so very many, including my work to advance women in sports and beyond.

In 1994, at the height of my career, I received a call from Yolanda Jackson, head of athlete engagement at the Women's Sports Foundation, which was founded in 1974 by tennis legend Billie Jean King. I was invited to attend the foundation's Annual Salute in New York City.

I was overwhelmed by the atmosphere of camaraderie, mutual respect, and professionalism. In addition to attending their gala, they offered free classes that empowered us as athletes to market ourselves, find sponsors, gain experience with the media, and educate us about the importance of continuing Billie Jean King's fight for all girls and women to have equitable access to sports across America. It was incredible to meet so many women athletes and to share our experiences with each other. All of us, no matter how big or small the sport, were treated like VIPs. It built our confidence and helped us want to step up and do more for our sport and do more for WSF. I was encouraged to participate on the foundation's committees, and on the board of trustees. At first, I was quite reluctant, with no confidence in my abilities. But with encouragement, I overcame that reluctance. I am so glad that I did. They did, and continue to do, an incredible job creating opportunities for girls and women and advocating for equity beyond such opportunities.

I served on the board from 2001 to 2006, for two consecutive three-year terms as the trustee of the foundation. From their inception to Title IX's 50th anniversary in 2022, WSF has invested over $100 million to expand access and opportunities for girls and women in sports. I was so blessed to be part of their effort to raise awareness of the importance of enforcing Title IX, so that our sisters and mothers and daughters can have as much access and opportunities to sports as their male counterparts.

> Title IX of the Education Amendments Act of 1972 is a federal law that states:
>
> "No person in the United States shall, on the basis of sex, be excluded from participation in, be denied the benefits of, or be subjected to discrimination under any education program or activity receiving federal financial assistance."

I'm sure I would never have had these incredibly enriching personal and professional opportunities without the assistance and influence of the Women's Sports Foundation.

The people there inspired me to be a fierce advocate for the organization, whose mission was to advance women in sports, and in life.

As I sit here in my Tampa home, thinking about all my accomplishments and achievements, and all those memories, writing the final words of this book, I stop for a moment. And I wonder.

How do you end your memoir? How do you know when you have told your entire life story the best that you can tell it?

I sit here, as I write these final words, feeling completely blessed. I know some people might question that. How can I feel blessed in the middle of a terminal cancer diagnosis?

I am blessed because of this wonderful life I have had, this amazing career I have had after walking into a pool hall in Manhattan at 18 years old.

I am blessed because in the far-back corner of that pool hall in 1989, I saw a guy creating geometrical magic at a green felt table, and I fell deeply and madly in love with the game.

I am blessed because I was an awkward, skinny, insecure girl fighting hellish scoliosis, who fought her way out of her shell. I am blessed because I became one of the most famous pool players of my time, which allowed me to empower women, Asian people, and those struggling with mental and physical disabilities, and now specifically women suffering with ovarian cancer, as they watched me battle it out in a man's sport.

> "With the current ascendance of women's sports, I am reminded that Jeanette was a forerunner for women in sports. Her contribution should not be forgotten."
>
> —John Skipper, former president of ESPN

I am blessed because I have three beautiful, smart daughters, an amazing son, and two wonderful stepdaughters, who have made me a grandmother of five: three girls and two boys. I am blessed because we still have close, meaningful relationships that I cherish, and they believe in me.

I am blessed because my pain, my health battles, and my struggles meant something. They meant something because they allowed me to be a force of light for others going through their own struggles.

> "Jeanette is the most admirable athlete I've ever read about, I've ever met, or I've ever known. She would have probably been the greatest women's pool player of all time, if not for scoliosis. She is a true inspiration."
>
> —Don Wardell,
> Lee's longtime physician and friend

I am blessed because those Bible verses my mom used to plaster on my door when I was a rebellious teen, causing me to go into fits of rage, now come back to me. Those verses about faith and the goodness of God. They are a comfort as I face a life where I have to ponder the end.

> "Yea, though I walk through the valley of the shadow of death, I will fear no evil: for thou art with me; thy rod and thy staff they comfort me.... Surely goodness and mercy shall follow me all the days of my life: and I will dwell in the house of the Lord forever."
>
> —Psalm 23

I am blessed because, not long ago, I was baptized in the ocean. I had been baptized as a baby, but never as an adult. As I played pool, as I had my children, as I was diagnosed with cancer, I thought about making that commitment to God. Shortly after I finished chemo and the doctors told me my cancer would never be in remission, I made my decision.

As I was submerged into the ocean, and as I was lifted back out again, I stood up, soaking wet, and refreshed. I felt a glorious sense of renewal and I raised my arms into the air in sweet victory, tears streaming down my face.

> "For Jeanette, it's not about pool now. It's about life or death. And she must win."
>
> —Doris Lee, Jeanette's sister

I am blessed because my success has given me a platform that others don't have as they battle cancer. I believe everything you go through in life is an opportunity to help and inspire others. You can be someone people pity, or you can be a fierce force they can look up to.

I decided to tell the world about my cancer in hopes of lifting others out of the darkness. I wanted my battle with cancer to have a greater purpose.

When I was introduced to the V Foundation through ESPN, I met its longtime board member, college basketball analyst and cancer fighter Dick Vitale. When I attended his gala, I was blown away by Dick's passion for cancer research, and I knew then that the foundation was a perfect fit for me.

The V Foundation for Cancer Research was founded by legendary basketball coach Jim Valvano with one goal, to achieve "Victory Over Cancer." Valvano died at the age of 47, following a nearly year-long battle with metastatic adenocarcinoma.

He died in April 1993, less than two months after his famous *ESPY* speech, in which he said the words that now lift the spirits of cancer patients around the world: "Don't give up. Don't ever give up."

Since its formation in 1993, the V Foundation has awarded more than $350 million in cancer research grants nationwide and has grown to become one of the premier supporters of cutting-edge cancer research.

I became a partner with the V Foundation as an ambassador. I am so honored and humbled to be part of that organization.

No one makes the choice to get cancer, but how you respond to the disease, how you choose to look at life, you do have that choice. I think that's something Jim Valvano really wanted to push through—you have a choice to try to love and connect with others, and to laugh, to cry, and to have hope.

The pages of those old family photo albums at my parents' house end, and they end before my story really ever begins.

There are no photos of me as The Black Widow, wearing edgy clothing and taking the billiards' world by storm. There are no photos of me standing with a gold medal at the World Games or being inducted into halls of fame. There are no photos of me in TV ads or walking the red carpet at the *ESPYs*. There are no photos of me now, in my fifties, sometimes weak, sometimes using a cane, and always still fighting to survive.

There are so many more photos that should be in that album, so many more stories to tell.

Throughout my life, I have been someone people felt sorry for, someone they envied, someone they abused, someone they taunted, someone they idolized, someone they deserted, and someone they loved.

Yet, I wrote my own story. And isn't it always better to write your own story, even if it's the hardest thing you'll ever have to do?

I can promise you this. When you write your own story and you fight the good fight, you are going to get so much more out of this beautiful life.

In the end, I have realized that my story is a simple one. It's a story of putting one foot in front of the other, of forging ahead even when it felt like I couldn't take another step. It's a story of being grateful, even when my life seemed hopeless. It's a story about persevering, a story about forgiving, a story about loving.

And my greatest hope is that my story was inspiring to you.

ACKNOWLEDGMENTS

I FOUND WRITING A BOOK about my life to be very difficult. I have been blessed with a long life full of exciting events, great success, and a whole lot of wonderful, amazing people. I am distressed that I have had to leave some great stories and so many interesting and loving friends out. The constraints of time and number of pages demand it. Yet, with the abundant love and help of so many who have been with me through thick and thin, I'm so happy this book is finally coming out.

I choose to start with God Almighty for being there my entire life, guiding me, protecting me, forgiving me, and loving me unconditionally. As faulty a Christian as I am, I will forever seek to do better in honoring You. Thank You for my salvation.

Next, I have to thank my friends, my partners and all the people associated with the American Poolplayers Association. The members, both nationally and in my Tampa franchise, are my people. The loyalty of the APA executives, the Bell and Hubbart families, Greg Fletcher, my guy Jason Bowman, Kevin Hinkebein, and Jeff Hayes was over-the-top remarkable and heartwarming. In my darkest hours, fighting cancer while COVID was ravaging both my business and theirs, their willingness to support me anyway *literally saved me.* How can you ever adequately thank someone for that?

Anthony and Stephanie Spano, you were my friends but quickly became my family. Thank you for your love and support, your time, and your generosity during a period when everything was in chaos. Having you become my partners in Tampa Bay APA became the best decision I ever made. You treated me and my girls like family, while growing our business into the best league in the world. Steph, I love my Love Chest to save sentimental cards and letters so I could be reminded how loved I am. Thank you for bringing me food and orchids and gifts for the girls, sharing fun times with me, and sometimes carrying us through the hard times. It means the world to me that my girls and I have you here as our Tampa family.

Similarly, my representatives at Octagon are stand-up professionals. Long after representing me ceased to be a revenue consideration, they continued to look out for me. Their president, Phil de Picciotto, and my team of Teddy Bloch, Alyssa Romano, Jason Weichelt, and Jennifer Keene (who made arrangements for my autobiography with Triumph Books) are clearly do-the-right-thing people. How lucky I am to be associated with them. You have all gone over the top for me and I'm very grateful.

I'll be forever grateful to Amsterdam Billiards Club, La Cue, and Howard Beach Billiard Club for believing in me as an amateur and sponsoring me in all of the local and regional competitions that gave me the edge when I was a rookie on the pro tour.

One of the things about being an individual athlete is that you have no team or league as a support mechanism. I am supremely fortunate to have a group of friends who have been totally selfless in their assistance, but have also been key contributors to my success. Barbara Wong, my first best friend, was my maid of honor—thank you for always believing in me and teaching me what it meant to be strong and brave.

You always encouraged me when I was starting pool and arguing with my mom all the time. You believed I could do anything and you always saw the best in me, even when I hadn't yet seen it myself. And I'll never forget the contribution you made when you heard I was sick. I don't know anyone that keeps herself busier, but you dropped everything and sacrificed so much to be here for me during the cancer battle.

My best friends, Dianna Stinger, Marc Wilson, and Marlene Wilson, all allowed me the joy of continuing to compete around the world throughout my career, yet still be with my new baby, Cheyenne, and later, Chloe and Savvy. Dianna, I don't know where to start with you. You've always been, and continue to be, one of my most trusted friends. You're the one who I've leaned on the most and the longest over the last 19 years, both as my personal assistant and as my most devoted and loyal friend. You also always seem to give the best advice, whether or not I wanted to hear it. You're one of the nicest, kindest people I've ever known and you made it your mission to do whatever you could to help me and be there for me no matter what.

Bob Carman, thank you so much for loving me the way you have. For teaching me the value of keeping things simple. Thank you for being my life coach *and* my billiards coach. Thank you for being my confidante, companion, and close friend as I learned the value of refining my stroke and focusing on my fundamentals and having a nice glass of red wine. Thank you for your patience and sharing your wisdom. Knowing you has given me new perspectives on life, family, home, and friendships. I'm always learning such valuable life lessons when I'm with you. I'm so thankful for the time we've had, especially you coming back to take care of me for every major surgery I've had, knowing I'd need the support. Or when you knew I needed someone to give me a hard time (lol). You've just loved me and understood me, probably better than anyone. It seems like something little, but for me, I've felt misunderstood my entire life, so it's a big deal that I feel like you see me. All of me. And I love you.

Thank you for introducing me to Jerry Briesath, whose world of knowledge was critical before winning the gold at the World Games.

Special thank you to Jerry Briesath and Mark Wilson for all the time, knowledge, and encouragement you've given me to become a more consistent player and equipped me with the tools to take my game to new heights.

Dr. Donald Wardell, thank you for practicing with me til all hours of the night, buying me Heath bars, reading bedtime stories to Cheyenne, being our doctor 24/7, helping at tournaments and my sales booth, showing us how real french toast is made, giving my presenter speech at my Hall of Fame induction, and even setting up shots for me and helping me gear up for competition. I'm so grateful to you for stepping up in every way, any time we needed you, since the day I met you—including medically—throughout our 20-year friendship. Thank you for being one of the closest fans, friends, teachers, and students I've ever had. I love you and appreciate you.

Gene, Shylee, Julie, you've spent the most time with me over the last five years here in Tampa. Gene, thank you for loving the girls and me, protecting us, having fun with us, spoiling us, and being an incredible father figure to the girls when they really needed it. Shylee, I watched you grow up before my eyes, from when you started assisting me in the league to becoming the league office manager and a young woman that I grew to respect, love, admire, trust, depend on, and truly want your dreams to come true. I'm so blessed to have been a part of your life. I've always believed in you, but now, as I watch you soar, I'm here, so proud of you, and will always consider you a daughter that I shall love deeply and forever.

Julie, geez, I don't know what I would've done without you. Really. Taking on running my league on my own was the hardest thing I ever had to do, and without you taking care of my house and the kids *and* me, there would have been no way for me to do my job. I love you, Julie. Thank you, now and forever.

My darling son John, Gabby, Jenny, Danny, and Marc all rushed to my side as I went through chemotherapy and stayed for three months. Who does that?! You guys were amazing and I'll never forget the time you took for me. For cleaning or fixing things in the house, tending to my girls with so much love, redoing all my girls' bedrooms with new paint and flooring, and stocking us with the best groceries and culinary meals *ever*! My girls Morgan and Olivia, Jeff, Kris, Dianna, and Bonnie, thank you for visiting as soon as you could. It meant so much to me, especially during COVID.

Rachel and Jin, my little sisters, thank you for coming to visit and taking care of me, my girls, and even taking time to help me purge my ridiculous Black Widow wardrobe closet. Marlene, I really wished we could've spent more time together, but we were all so glad to see you. You're their second mom after all. Thank you for taking care of us and for cleaning the whole house! Whew. I know that was a lot.

Don, Jeff, and Barbara, thank you for your generosity and renting those beachfront condos for us to get out of our self-quarantine and enjoy some privacy and sunshine. Others that stepped up to do whatever they could remotely on multiple occasions were my sister, Doris; cousins Jessica, Esther, and Liza; and friends Kathy Hawk, Lisa Just, Delbert Wong, Janet Atwell, Kris Moran, Jeremy and Kim Jones, Stu Mattana, and Legends of Pocket Billiards.

Doris, I'm so grateful that you're my big sister. I'm so glad you reached out to me in my twenties and made the effort to reconnect. Even when I was hesitant to respond, you never gave up and, because of that, I have a big sister that I can talk to, get advice from, and share memories with in a way that no one else can. No one in the world but you would've done the work you did when you came to take care of me and help me in the way that you did. Thank you for being there to help whenever I need you, especially since cancer. Although it must have been so tough on you, you hung in to be there for me, us, even when I was awful to you at times.

Thank you, Tom, Doris, Dianna, Liza, and Kris for helping me keep up with messages and mail and any admin stuff that I needed to take care of when I couldn't any longer. I'm so thankful for how generous you were with your time, when I know you had your own busy lives. It takes a village sometimes.

Esther, you really can't imagine what a role you've played in my life. As a kid, you were my best (and only) close friend. We did everything together. You were my little sidekick. But through the years, I've seen you mature in the most beautiful way into a woman I look up to, who is so kind, considerate, flattering, funny, sweet, witty, generous, and an incredibly loving and attentive mom who sacrifices everything for her family in a way that I know makes God so proud. You made God the center of your life for as long as I can remember and Esther, you have godly children that are just like you. I don't know how anyone can do better than that. I really look up to you as a friend, cousin, mother, and as a woman. Anyone is lucky to have you in their life. Thank you for hosting me all the years I would travel to New York, going out of your way to spoil me as though I was a star, but not because of it. You are just that loving to everyone, but you make us all feel so special when you're the one that's so special. I'm also thankful to you, Jin, and my darlings, Lauren, Daniel, Audrey, Michael, and Kathleen, for feeding all of us home-cooked meals, playing games with my girls, and treating me as a recovering patient with VIP level of care and attention.

To Jeannie Seaver and Sonya Chbeeb, thank you so much for helping and supporting me. James and Liza, thank you so much for moving here to assist us. Danny, I can't thank you enough for living with us over the last 18 months, to help me and the girls in a way no one else could. I can't thank you enough for completely putting your life on hold just to be there for us.

Mike Panozzo and Mike Howerton from *Billiards Digest* and *AZ Billiards*, thank you so much for covering my journey, helping me tell my story, and assisting Tom in promoting the GoFundMe campaign.

Our God has blessed me with a large supportive and understanding family. It is not easy to have a globetrotting celebrity Mom, but my remarkable kids made it work. Morgan and Jason, Olivia and Ben, John and Taylor, Cheyenne, Chloe, and Savannah, I'm so proud of you and I love each of you so much. My beautiful grandkids, Ellie, Lijah, Bash, and Nori, I love you too, so much! My love for you, and you for me, gave me the will and courage to fight.

Also, I wanted to separate out two people in a special way, Dana Benbow and Tom George...

Dana, from the start, I liked you enough that I thought we'd become good lifelong friends but, as our time went on, I realized you were meant to be my angel. Few people are as smart, talented, considerate, and loving as you, but far fewer are as selfless, open-minded, accepting, inspiring, constantly encouraging, and understanding. You never, ever made me feel judged for being the way that I am and always made time for me. You were so patient with me, worked around my schedule, and made it clear that you were willing to do whatever it took to make this a book something of which I would be supremely proud. But through all of that, you captured my voice! You wanted this so badly *for me*, for *my sake*, and I truly believe you were exactly the right person to help me write my story. I will cherish you and my memoir forever because of it.

Tom, how do you measure the value of having someone in your life who always believes in you, who you trust implicitly, whose advice you respect? Your hard work, integrity, perseverance, and intelligence through the decades have earned my trust. Even if you were blessed enough to know someone like that, could they and would they stop everything to sacrifice full time to make sure that you have the freedom and the means to enjoy the blessings of life with those most precious to you, for the remainder of whatever time you have left? Only you. When you call, my phone screen reads, "My HERO Literally," because in my darkest hour, as soon as you heard, you drove six hours to sit with me in person, with a tablet and pen, and said, "What can I do to help?" From that point forward, three years later, you have dedicated your time to doing everything you could, to give me time with family and help me fill my emotional need to find platforms, like this book and becoming an ambassador for the V Foundation, so that my experiences can help others suffering with cancer. Even now, you're still doing everything you can to help me tell my story and to help me make an income for my family so I don't worry too much. I can't remember how many times you told me to relax and quit worrying. Stress is terrible for cancer! That's easy to say, but you make it possible. Tom, thank you for being my HERO, for continuing to dedicate your life to making my dreams come true, for putting up with me during my bad days and creating and celebrating so many of my greatest ones. I am so intensely grateful and I love you, always.

To all my fans, I am "The Black Widow" because of *you*. Your love and support made me possible. Thank you now and forever.

—Jeanette Lee
March 2024